# Measurement of patients' satisfaction with their care

Edited by

**Ray Fitzpatrick**
*Fellow, Nuffield College & University Lecturer in Medical Sociology, University of Oxford*

and

**Anthony Hopkins**
*Director, Research Unit, Royal College of Physicians*

1993

ROYAL COLLEGE OF PHYSICIANS OF LONDON

**Royal College of Physicians of London**
**11 St Andrews Place, London NW1 4LE**

**Registered Charity No. 210508**

Copyright © 1993 Royal College of Physicians of London
ISBN 1 873240 53 8

Typeset by Dan-Set Graphics, Telford, Shropshire
Printed in Great Britain by Cathedral Print Services Ltd,
Rollestone Street, Salisbury SP1 1DX

# Foreword

**by Leslie Turnberg**
*President, Royal College of Physicians*

Advances in medicine are occurring at a rapid rate and, with the increasingly technological approach to investigation and treatment, doctors naturally focus on the need to carry them out competently and safely. In doing so, however, some may overlook the very real need to listen to their patients, to explore their concerns and to explain what they propose. The College, recognising the need for better communication between patients and all health professionals, has set up a Working Party on Communication, which will publish its findings.

Physicians also need to explain what outcomes may be realistically achieved by their interventions—the likely prognosis. Unfortunately, it is sometimes difficult to make any real impact upon the underlying disease. In these circumstances in particular, patients value a physician's support; they also wish to feel that their physicians have understood their individual concerns. Patient satisfaction is itself therefore an outcome of health care and, like any other outcome, requires measurement. Although the College welcomes the government's initiative in the publication of *The Patient's Charter*, it believes that such aspects as waiting times in outpatients and attractiveness of accommodation are only one aspect of the provision of health care about which patients may express their satisfaction or dissatisfaction. More important is the development of measures of satisfaction with what physicians and other health professionals do in the course of their daily clinical work to try to relieve patients. In this book, Ray Fitzpatrick, of Nuffield College, Oxford, and Anthony Hopkins, Director of the College's Research Unit, bring together some of their own work and the work of colleagues in developing sensitive, reliable and valid measures which have been adequately researched.

I believe this book should help all those concerned with the needs of patients—doctors as well as others—in their efforts to improve health care. It demonstrates further the College's commitment to professional standards and the quality of medical care.

L.A.T.

# Contributors

**Richard H. Baker,** *Director, Eli Lilly National Medical Audit Centre, Department of General Practice, Leicester General Hospital, Gwendolen Road, Leicester LE5 4PW.*

**Ray Fitzpatrick,** *Fellow, Nuffield College & University Lecturer in Medical Sociology, Department of Public Health and Primary Care, University of Oxford.*

**Cathy Gritzner,** *Research Manager (PATSAT), CASPE Research, King Edward's Hospital Fund for London, 14 Palace Court, London W2 4HT.*

**Anthony Hopkins,** *Director, Research Unit, Royal College of Physicians, 11 St Andrews Place, London NW1 4LE.*

**Linda Lamont,** *Director, The Patients Association, 18 Victoria Park Square, Bethnal Green, London E2 9PF.*

**Ralph Leavey,** *Senior Lecturer, School of Health, St Martin's College, Lancaster LA1 3JD.*

**Michael Pryce-Jones,** *Management Consultant, The Oxford Consultancy, Oxford Regional Services Consortium, Old Road, Headington, Oxford OX3 7LF.*

**Andrew G. H. Thompson,** *Lecturer in Quantitative Methods, Cardiff Business School, University of Wales, Aberconway Building, Colum Drive, Cardiff CF1 3EU.*

**Alison J. Wilson,** *Freelance Research Worker.*

# Contents

# Members of the Workshop (in alphabetical order)

**Richard H. Baker**, *The Leckhampton Surgery, Cheltenham*

**Clare Bradley**, *Senior Lecturer in Psychology, Royal Holloway and Bedford New College, Egham*

**Jocelyn Cornwell**, *Audit Commission, London*

**June M. Crown**, *Head of Public Health, Institute of Public Health, Tunbridge Wells*

**Ray Fitzpatrick**, *Lecturer in Medical Sociology, Nuffield College, Oxford*

**\*Terence Geffen**, *Specialist in Community Medicine, North West Thames Regional Health Authority, London*

**Cathy Gritzner**, *Research Manager, CASPE Research, King Edward's Hospital Fund for London, London*

† **Mark Harrison**, *Consultant Urological Surgeon, Royal Hampshire County Hospital, Winchester*

**Anthony Hopkins**, *Director, Research Unit, Royal College of Physicians, London*

**Danny Kelly**, *Research Assistant, Department of Medical Sociology, Nuffield College, Oxford*

**Zarrina Kurtz**, *Regional Paediatric Epidemiologist, South West Thames Regional Health Authority, London*

**Linda Lamont**, *Director, The Patients Association, London*

**Shirley McKiber**, *Quality Improvement Programme, King's Fund Centre for Health Services Development, London*

**Duncan Macpherson**, *Senior Medical Officer, Department of Health, London*

**Michael Pryce-Jones**, *Management Consultant, The Oxford Consultancy, Oxford*

**Debbie Sandford**, *Audit Commission, London*

† **Veronica Sowton**, *Business Manager Outpatients, Royal Hampshire County Hospital, Winchester*

**Jackie Spiby**, *Consultant in Public Health, Beckenham*

**Andrew G. H. Thompson**, *Lecturer in Quantitative Methods, Cardiff Business School, University of Wales, Cardiff*

**Paul Walker**, *Director of Public Health, Norwich District Health Authority, Norwich*

**David Wilkin**, *Deputy Director, Centre for Primary Care Research, University of Manchester, Rusholme Health Centre, Manchester*

**Alison J. Wilson**, *North Manchester Community Drugs Team, Manchester*

\* At the workshop Dr Geffen presented a paper on *'Patient complaints as a means of understanding dissatisfaction with care'*

† Mr Harrison and Mrs Sowton presented a paper on *'A management perspective'*, jointly written with Dr D. J. Hewett, Director of Public Health, Winchester Health Authority

*Copies of these papers are available from the College Publications Office on request*

# 1 | Scope and measurement of patient satisfaction

**Ray Fitzpatrick**
*Department of Public Health and Primary Care,
University of Oxford*

Evaluation of the quality of health care has emerged as a key issue for all health services, and for some time it has been recognised that the patient's views are an essential component of such evaluations. Thus Doll argued that the National Health Service (NHS) should be evaluated in terms of three distinct criteria: medical outcomes, economic efficiency and social acceptability;[1] the last is an alternative expression for patient satisfaction. Similarly Maxwell distinguishes six dimensions by which the quality of health care may be assessed: access, relevance to need, effectiveness, equity, efficiency and social acceptability.[2] Other recent discussions of quality of health care also include this component.[3,4] However, unease is often expressed about the proper role, scope and validity of patients' contributions to assessing the quality of health care. It is right therefore that a volume should be devoted to examining the measurement issues surrounding patient satisfaction. This book presents a range of methods that may be used to assess the patient's views about his or her health care.

The term 'patient satisfaction' is widely used, but it is seldom defined and almost never theoretically examined.[5] Amongst the few attempts to clarify the concept, Pascoe regards satisfaction as a health care recipient's reaction to salient aspects of his or her experience of service.[6] Satisfaction involves a *cognitive evaluation* of and an *emotional reaction* to health care. Linder-Pelz similarly argues that patient satisfaction involves the expression of an *attitude* and *evaluation* in relation to health care.[7] Both observations contrast patient satisfaction with patients' reports of more objective aspects of their care, such as the length of time they have waited for an appointment.[8] There is a strong tradition in the United Kingdom (UK) of using patient surveys to examine areas such as length of time waiting at the surgery or availability of home visits from the doctor, in which patients provide basic information about the nature of their health care as well as subjective evaluations of their care.[9,10]

Measurements or assessments of patient satisfaction have been employed in a number of different contexts by users with similar but not identical purposes. At least three parallel developments have occurred in the use of surveys of patients' views. The first and most dominant application in this country has been managerially led. An enormous number of local surveys have been conducted during the past few years, largely sponsored by health authorities with regard to hospital, community and primary care services.[11] This approach received strong impetus from the Griffiths report on NHS management which found fault with the NHS for failing to obtain and act on feedback from its customers.[12] The more recent White Paper by the Secretary of State for Health, *Working for patients*,[13] reinforced the need for health authorities to improve the quality of services by taking more systematic account of users' views. This first approach, whilst being important in putting the assessment of patient satisfaction clearly on the agenda of health authorities, has largely focused on areas of health services amenable to managerial intervention, for example physical amenities and 'hotel' aspects of care. Areas such as clinical activity and outcomes of health care are currently considered to be contentious subjects for managerial involvement.

A second strand in the development of measures of patient satisfaction has been their use in more formal and systematic health services research, particularly in addressing questions regarding the organisation and delivery of health care. Measures of patient satisfaction have been used to examine patients' perceptions of alternative forms of paying for health care,[14] and alternative forms of management of medical problems, especially in the USA.[15] In such applications, patient satisfaction is used, usually alongside other outcomes, systematically to address a specific question. The most rigorous use of such techniques has been the RAND health insurance experiment in which a randomised prospective design was used to evaluate the costs and consequences of alternative health plans.[16] As part of this study Davies, Ware and colleagues developed measures of patient satisfaction to examine consumers' views.[17] To date, health services research has not been as well developed in the UK, and satisfaction measures have been less frequently used, especially in such elaborate forms as the RAND experiment. However, Cartwright and colleagues have a long record of using surveys of patients' views as a key resource in examining hospital and primary care services.[9,10]

Although of interest to clinical practice, neither of the two areas of development discussed so far has emerged with a specifically clinical focus. The third area examines the role of patient satisfaction in relation to the content of medical care, and is of most relevance to this book. A disparate body of studies has begun to appear across a wide range of fields of health care. Thus patients' views have been measured with regard to their treatment for specific conditions such as diabetes,[18] back pain,[19] cancer,[20] congestive heart failure[21] and sexually transmitted diseases.[22] More common than such condition-specific studies have been investigations into how the medical consultation and patterns of communication affect outcomes such as satisfaction and adherence to medical advice both in hospital practice[23] and in primary care.[24]

Although all three approaches are equally interested in the assessment of patients' views, the degree of attention to measurement issues has differed somewhat in the three fields. At one extreme, health authorities and management often set out to assess patient satisfaction with fairly simple ambitions. The main purpose is to identify problems in the provision of care that may be improved by managerial intervention. Their main method is to obtain descriptive accounts of levels of satisfaction with different aspects of health care included in the survey. This kind of feedback can actually be obtained equally well by methods other than the conventional structured survey, for example by patient participation groups, public meetings, advisory groups, and qualitative market research methods.[11,25,26] At the other extreme, university-based health services research sets out with the more ambitious objective of using patient satisfaction to answer questions in a more definitive way.[16] The results are expected to be of general scientific importance. More emphasis therefore tends to be placed on establishing the measurement properties of instruments, and on demonstrating statistical relationships between patient satisfaction and relevant aspects of health care. The differences between these two approaches might be exaggerated, and they have different agenda, and different time horizons and available resources.

Patient satisfaction as assessed in clinical research sits somewhere in the middle of this spectrum. In principle, the medical profession might be expected to adopt the more formal approach of health services research, for example by requiring such levels of reliability in measurement as are expected (but not always found) in clinical or laboratory methods.[27] However, in the more practical context of medical audit, the degree of attention and level of resources available mean that compromises may have to be made in relation to the design and measurement capabilities of satisfaction questionnaires.

The view that patient satisfaction is an important dimension of the quality of health care can be seen to be more than rhetorical in the light of the growing body of research. Two kinds of evidence are briefly examined. First, it is clear that patient satisfaction is related to other important outcomes of health care. Second, patient satisfaction is related to a number of aspects of how the clinician interacts with his or her patient.

## Patient satisfaction in relation to other outcomes

A number of studies have found that patients who are more satisfied with their experiences of health care are more likely to follow the advice they receive or adhere to medical regimes. Evidence comes from studies of outpatient clinics in paediatrics[23] and neurology,[28] as well as from research in general practice.[29,30] Dissatisfied patients are more likely to fail to reattend,[31,32] to change their doctor or health plan,[16,33,34] or resort to unorthodox medicine.[35]

A number of studies indicate that patient satisfaction is related to outcomes in terms of health status.[18,19,36–42] In all these studies, poorer health status is associated with higher dissatisfaction. In some instances health status is the strongest predictor of satisfaction.[43] There are a number of possible explanations for such findings. It may be that those with long-term poorer health are inclined to view a number of aspects of their lives negatively, including the quality of their health care. In this case satisfaction scores may not actually reflect quality of care. An alternative is that those with poorer long-term health receive a less satisfactory standard of care. Health care professionals may not find the care of patients with long-term poor health as rewarding as that of the acutely ill, especially if poorer health status is associated with psychological distress. This response on the part of health professionals may be detected by patients and ultimately reflected in higher dissatisfaction.[37,44] This second explanation suggests that associations between dissatisfaction and poorer health status are evidence of real differences in the quality of care. In many studies it is difficult to establish the direction of causation. However, in a few studies satisfaction is predictive of subsequent improvements in health.[19,36] These studies suggest the possibility that satisfaction may influence health status rather than the reverse. Hall and colleagues suggest two intervening mechanisms for such a relationship.[37] One possibility is that, as established by a number of studies, satisfied patients are more likely to follow the doctor's medical advice, which in turn gives the treatment more chance to have beneficial effect. The second possibility is that some placebo form of non-specific benefit may be responsible. In a study of neurological management of headache in which satisfaction did predict symptomatic improvement one year later, patients' detailed comments suggested that the sense of being understood and having their health problem taken seriously may well have had such non-specific therapeutic effects[36] (Chapter 6).

**Patient satisfaction in relation to interpersonal skills**

Surveys have indicated that doctors' interpersonal skills have a substantial influence on patients' overall levels of satisfaction with doctors' care.[45] Patient satisfaction is higher with doctors whose empathic skills have independently been shown to be greater.[46] The ability to take a medical history in a way that encourages patients to express their own views about the problem is similarly related to patient satisfaction.[47] Discovering patients' main concerns and expectations[23] and being able to conduct a consultation that involves the patient in a more active sense have also been found to be positively related to satisfaction.[48] Appropriate and comprehensible information[49] and effective reassurance[36] are other important influences upon satisfaction. Patient satisfaction data have also been used to show that patients appreciate consultations that give sufficient time to address their problems.[50] In primary care, continuity of care also has a large effect upon patient satisfaction[51] (see also Chapter 8).

The significance of the evidence listed in the preceding paragraph is that in nearly all instances significant relationships between satisfaction and *independent* measures of specific aspects of the consultation have been found, usually by audio or video recordings of consultations which are then systematically rated by independent observers. The aspects of consultations found to influence outcomes such as satisfaction are consistent with patient-centred models of training in communication skills which are increasingly being emphasised in medical education.[52]

**Patient satisfaction as a multidimensional construct**

The search for a single answer to the question of whether a patient is satisfied with his or her health care is misconceived. As with

**Table 1.** Different dimensions of patient satisfaction.

|  |  |
|---|---|
| • Humaneness | • Cost |
| • Informativeness | • Facilities |
| • Overall quality | • Health outcome |
| • Competence | • Continuity |
| • Bureaucracy | • Attention to psychosocial problems |
| • Access | |

Adapted from Hall and Dornan, 1988 (reference 53).

other areas of health services research, such as quality of life and subjective health status, patient satisfaction has proved to be a multidimensional construct. Single global scores may therefore disguise divergent judgements on different aspects of care. Overall, patients may hold quite distinct views with regard to the technical, interpersonal and amenity aspects of their health care. Cleary and McNeil delineated nine different dimensions that contribute to patient satisfaction: the art of care, technical quality, accessibility, convenience, finance, physical environment, availability, continuity and outcome.[8] A similar list of specific aspects of care that may be distinguished in patients' judgements of satisfaction is provided by Hall and Dornan (Table 1).[53] Correlations between different dimensions are often high, and the effects of different aspects of care upon overall satisfaction are not easily detected. It has been suggested that there are particularly powerful halo effects involved in patients' judgements about health care; in particular, strong impressions of the personal qualities of a doctor (with regard to 'humaneness' or 'art of care') may shape other judgements made, for example, with regard to the value or technical competence of care received.[54] Some studies have suggested that patients form one single attitude with regard to their doctor's conduct, in which judgements of elements of technical competence and quality are indistinguishable from judgements of humaneness (such as consideration and support).[55] However, other studies, both qualitative[56] and quantitative,[57] indicate that respondents are capable of making refined and distinctive judgements about different aspects of their care.

A technical problem with such multidimensional instruments arises if a summary score is wanted. A common solution is simply to add the scores of the different dimensions, thereby giving equal weight to different aspects. Thus the Client Satisfaction Questionnaire, intended to be applicable in a wide range of service settings, in its most commonly used version has 18 questionnaire items covering a diverse range of areas (comfort and attractiveness of physical setting, promptness of service, staff understanding of problem etc).[58] Each item has four possible answers, and individuals' answers are then summed to produce a range of scores from 18 to 72. This solution makes too strong an assumption about the equal importance of different areas of health care, and does not make it easy to detect contrary trends between dimensions (for example, patients satisfied with staff interpersonal skills but dissatisfied with accessibility). For these reasons it is recommended that dimensions be kept separate in analysis, as in other health care evaluation instruments.[59] A third solution, which has not been attempted with any instruments developed in the UK, has been to weight different items, either by deriving weights from judgements of lay panels or by incorporating respondents' judgements of the importance of different scales.[53] The results of such exercises may reduce the intuitive meaning and appeal of simpler systems.

Understanding of the significance of different dimensions has developed at different rates. Measures in the areas of interpersonal care, communication and humaneness have been used with particular success to tease out the relationship between aspects of medical consultations and their effects on satisfaction.[48] Other dimensions (particularly satisfaction with health outcomes) are far less frequently measured, so we have less understanding of how they are affected by processes of care.[8,53] A meta-analysis of a largely American series of patient satisfaction studies found that the dimensions of care most frequently included were humaneness, informativeness, overall quality and competence,[53] whereas the dominant themes of UK studies appear to be dimensions related to amenity, a contrast that may indicate the greater integration of managerial and medical concerns in the USA.

**Issues of measurement in relation to patient satisfaction**

At the core of the concept of patient satisfaction are some issues of measurement which have been frequently rehearsed but barely resolved. One fundamental problem is that results from patient satisfaction surveys produce little variation, with most respondents expressing positive satisfaction. There are a number of different possible explanations for this tendency, but one factor undoubtedly is that patients are reluctant to express criticism of the NHS or of health professionals—so-called 'normative effects'.[56] The extent of positive skew in patient satisfaction surveys may be overstated.

One of the most comprehensive reviews to date, a meta-analysis of published patient satisfaction surveys,[53] concluded that the mean score across surveys, if results were standardised to a range of 0–1.00, was 0.76. Expressed another way, the mean proportion of positively satisfied respondents was 81%. Such skewed distributions undoubtedly pose basic problems in the analysis and interpretation of survey results, especially when the sample is small. However, it should be of major concern to those providing health services that, despite normative effects limiting expression of critical comment, about one in five patients may be expected to be dissatisfied with some aspects of their care.

Many of the developments of measurement in this field stem largely from this initial problem of limited variation and normative effects. Thus questionnaires are designed to encourage more varied responses by, for example, offering graded responses to questionnaire items, or choices of response that reflect more natural ways in which respondents might talk about their health care (eg reference 60). Chapters 2 and 5 emphasise the iterative process required in the construction of questionnaires; one of the factors involved when choosing which questionnaire items should be eliminated is evidence of a highly skewed distribution of answers.

Ware and Hays carried out one of the few systematic studies to examine variation in patient satisfaction.[61] They examined the effects of two alternative forms of response. On four different dimensions of satisfaction, patients expressed their views either by means of six choices ranging from 'extremely satisfied' to 'very dissatisfied' or by means of a five-choice scale from 'excellent' to 'fair'. The second format was repeatedly found to produce more variation in patients' responses, and was also better at predicting intentions to return to the same doctor and comply with medical advice. They also noted that the positioning of satisfaction items in the questionnaire as a whole made a significant difference to variation. When satisfaction items followed rather than preceded other items of a more factual nature, patients gave more varied answers. It is possible that the more factual items led patients to more considered appraisal of their treatment experiences.

Other aspects of satisfaction questionnaires are designed specifically to overcome the problem when respondents give socially acceptable answers; confidentiality of replies and neutrality of data gatherers must be guaranteed.

A second problem is the effect of social, demographic and other variables upon responses. With the exception of age, older patients invariably reporting more satisfaction, such background factors appear to be inconsistent in effects between studies.[37,53] Other variables that may influence responses include gender, educational level, and the ethnic group to which the patient belongs. One particular problem is that effects of demographic variables upon satisfaction are prone to vary depending on the influence of moderating variables. Thus one study showed that men are more satisfied than women with health care amongst ethnic minorities but not amongst whites.[53] Often the details of surveys are under-reported, so it is hard to put together an overview of such effects. It remains unclear whether such effects are due to real differences in health care experiences or to differences in expectations or ways of responding to questionnaires.[8] It is possible to allow for the influence of social characteristics by sub-group analysis of the data. A particular challenge to the interpretation of satisfaction surveys is the growing evidence that poorer health status is related to dissatisfaction (Chapter 8). The available evidence could be consistent with quite different causal explanations of this relationship. The most important general point is the need to examine the results of satisfaction surveys for artifacts producd by effects of background variables, especially when comparing two or more population samples or following changes over time. Any differences in satisfaction scores obtained between two or more hospital units or general practices may be due to simple differences in patient characteristics.

The third problem is one common to all measuring instruments, the establishment of how well questionnaires and interviews measure accurately patient satisfaction. One aspect of the question is reliability—whether the instrument produces the same results on repeated use under the same conditions. This is conventionally examined either by inspecting stability over repeated administration of the questionnaire (*test–retest reliability*) or considering the consistency of items tapping a single concept (*internal reliability*).

One of the earliest studies to examine test–retest reliability of a patient satisfaction instrument produced quite encouraging results.[23] Retesting may give a misleading impression of reliability if the standard statistic of a correlation coefficient is used, because this may miss the phenomenon of the sample as a whole shifting its level of satisfaction. It is by no means easy to interpret such shifts. For example, a general practice study found a significant reduction in levels of satisfaction between assessment immediately after a consultation and just one week later.[24] It is difficult to determine whether such changes are an indication of the poor reliability of instruments or of underlying changes in satisfaction.

To avoid such difficulties, surveys are more likely to look at a more manageable aspect of reliability—internal reliability, the internal agreement of items, by which criterion a number of instruments emerge as satisfactory. Ware and Hays review a number of scales from patient satisfaction instruments that have reliability coefficients exceeding 0.90.[61]

It is common for views about patient satisfaction in the USA to be assessed by means of Likert scales. Individuals are asked to state to what extent they agree with each of a number of statements. The items within a scale are summed and the total is the individual's score for that construct. Usually such scales have required prior testing to eliminate items unrelated to the construct of interest, and to establish that items do correlate with each other to a satisfactory extent. Resort to scales instead of individual questionnaire items has occurred not only because of formal psychometric evidence that scales more accurately measure underlying attitudes[62] but also because of the increased range of scores that is obtained. Chapter 5 illustrates this approach.

The *validity* of a patient satisfaction instrument is more difficult to establish. Effort has to be put into examining validity because, as Baker observes in Chapter 5, health professionals are unlikely to change their behaviour in the light of evidence that they cannot believe. The most practical approach is to examine whether the contents of instruments appear to cover clearly and unambiguously the full scope of what it is intended that they measure (*content validity*). Individuals with as diverse a range of backgrounds as possible should be involved in this phase of the development of instruments to ensure that all aspects may be covered, as is the best practice in the field of measurement of quality of life.[63] Lay people should be included in the earliest stages of design of satisfaction instruments.[64] This is often achieved by exploratory pilot surveys using open-ended methods of interview to maximise the range of issues raised by patients. Pilot versions of questionnaires can leave space at the end in which respondents are invited to comment on subjects not otherwise addressed. More formal methods of examining the validity of satisfaction instruments have been used. Thus *construct validity* can be used to examine whether satisfaction scores relate to processses of care that have been independently measured.[65] Leavey and Wilson examine in Chapter 4 the consistency within their primary care questionnaires of different items, for example between the reported length of time required to obtain an appointment and acceptability of this delay. *Convergent validity* and *divergent validity* similarly address the question of whether satisfaction instruments produce sensible patterns of agreement and disagreement within an array of other variables. The principle involved here is that items should correlate most with items to which, in theoretical terms, they are similar and least with items from which they are most distant. An overall matrix of correlations can then be presented.[19,66]

The most demanding of all criteria is *criterion validity*—instruments are assessed against an accepted external criterion. It might be argued that there cannot be any 'gold standard' against which to judge the views of patients. Nevertheless an interesting application of this approach is provided in Chapter 5 by Baker. Scores for patients' views about their primary care are examined against the criterion of external judges' assessments of the same practices (Chapter 5). There have been a few other studies that relate patient satisfaction scores to independent assessments: for example, of the interpersonal skills and technical proficiency of health professionals.[66] However, it must be remembered that the main point of assessing patients' judgements is that they provide a distinct and different perspective about the quality of health care, so external criteria may not really be appropriate.

Again practical constraints make such methods beyond the scope of most who intend to obtain the views of patients. They are more likely to rely either on content validity or on the more general advice, applicable to all surveys, that questionnaire items should be as precise and specific as possible, and above all should be piloted and checked for intelligibility, acceptability and capacity to generate variation.

**Methods of data collection**

There is a wide choice of methods available to obtain the views of patients. The fixed format, self-completed questionnaire is most frequently used for obvious reasons of economy and ease of administration and processing. The format also imposes standardisation of data. It is sometimes also observed that the questionnaire eliminates problems of 'interviewer bias', but in reality this is not a problem when trained interviewers are used. Undoubtedly interviews are more capable of permitting clarification of misunderstandings, exploring more complex views, establishing the reasons behind respondents' views, and providing graphic illustrative material. However, it is possible to overestimate the sensitivity of interviews compared with questionnaires. Whilst less responsive to respondents' priorities and concerns, a well piloted questionnaire should be well enough designed to encompass most dimensions of a problem. Now that patient satisfaction questionnaires have been successfully used to predict the patient's probability of changing his or her health care plan[33] or to distinguish physicians with greater or lesser interpersonal skills,[46] it should not be felt that the questionnaire is automatically second best in terms of sensitivity combined with practicality. There are several kinds of questionnaire format illustrated in this book, the common denominator being that careful development work has gone into establishing the intelligibility, acceptability and psychometric properties of the items in the questionnaire.

There are now various types of interview in use to assess patient satisfaction. The structured interview is closest in format to a personally administered questionnaire in that the interviewer keeps very close to a fixed set and format of questions. Its main advantages are clarification of items and respondent adherence. However, in many respects it is an expensive way of obtaining the information obtained almost as well by a self-completed questionnaire. To maximise respondents' candid expression of personal views, two other approaches appear similar in form and intention—the non-schedule standardised interview (used in Chapter 6 by Fitzpatrick and Hopkins) and interviews based on critical incident technique (discussed by Pryce-Jones in Chapter 7). Both attempt to encourage respondents as much as possible to report experiences and evaluations in their own terms. In both cases this is achieved by allowing the patient to tell a narrative of his or her experiences from which the interviewer is particularly interested to record positive and negative reactions. Both methods consume time and labour as they require personal interviews conducted by trained interviewers. It also takes a lot of time to analyse the results obtained at non-schedule standardised interviews as ratings of positive and negative comments have to be made. The advantage of non-schedule standardised interviews is that the results can be produced in quantitative format, and satisfaction can be related to specific aspects of patients' experiences by conventional multivariate analysis. An advantage of critical incident technique is that positive and negative comments are the main substance of feedback to staff. These may have a direct intuitive impact that survey reports often lack.

## Practical considerations

Consideration has to be given to how data regarding patients' views are to be gathered and processed, and how they are to be fed back into the health care system. It is essential to obtain views that are broadly representative of the relevant patient group. The precise nature of the relevant group will depend on the question being asked. The group may, for example, variously consist of all the patients who are treated in a particular ward or clinic, all the patients on a practice list, whether or not they have recently attended, or all individuals in a geographical area in a particular age group. Views that are representative may be achieved by attempting a census of all of the relevant group; this is the CASPE approach. More commonly some sampling strategy is used which, because of the practical constraints of health care settings, can rarely be truly random but usually can approach this requirement.[67]

The response rate is as important as the sampling strategy when evaluating the representative nature of survey results. Chapter 3 shows that CASPE surveys have produced only modest response rates. This may in part be due to delivering questionnaires impersonally via the internal hospital mail. Delivery by hand, combined with personal follow-up of non-respondents, can considerably increase the response rates.[68] Chapter 4 reviews the different strategies that may be used to increase the response rates of postal surveys.

Finally, thought has to be given to the ways in which results are to be fed back to the health care system. At one extreme, results may be disseminated via scientific publications. However, the conventional survey report may not be the most appropriate vehicle for the local use of satisfaction data for audit purposes. Chapter 3 describes some of the work of the CASPE group which has paid particular attention to the question of feedback. The results of questionnaires are machine-read and linked to the hospital information system. Standardised scores are presented to relevant units or wards in a format that compares results with both previous performance and the scores of other units. Evidence is also presented of practical changes that have resulted from such 'user friendly' feedback. This reflects the principles of audit—the identification of problems, the implementation of change, and the evaluation of the effects of change.

However, as has been emphasised, much of the focus of surveys such as those of CASPE has been on areas of health care such as catering, the physical environment, noise etc which may be identified fairly clearly by current survey methodology and which are also likely to be responsive to action by managers. It is not yet clear that the same methods of collection and feedback of data are as appropriate for more clinical areas of health care, where the underlying issues may be more complex, the indications for areas

requiring change less precise, and clinical behaviour less likely to
be altered so rapidly in the light of evidence of this kind. Whilst
the development of efficient technologies for assessing and processing patient-based data has been impressive, their implications
and relevance for core areas of professional behaviour have yet to
be explored.

## References

1. Doll R. Monitoring the National Health Service. *Proceedings of the Royal Society of Medicine.* 1973; **66:** 729–40.
2. Maxwell R. Quality assessment in health. *British Medical Journal* 1984; **288:** 1470–2.
3. Donabedian A. The quality of care: how can it be assessed? *Journal of the American Medical Association* 1988; **260:** 1743–8.
4. Hopkins A. *Measuring the quality of medical care.* London: RCP Publications, 1990.
5. Locker D, Dunt D. Theoretical and methodological issues in sociological studies of consumer satisfaction with medical care. *Social Science and Medicine* 1978; **12:** 283–92.
6. Pascoe G. Patient satisfaction in primary care: a literature review and analysis. *Evaluation and Program Planning* 1983; **6:** 185–210.
7. Linder-Pelz S. Toward a theory of patient satisfaction. *Social Science and Medicine* 1982; **16:** 577–82.
8. Cleary P, McNeil B. Patient satisfaction as indicator of quality of care. *Inquiry* 1988; **25:** 25–36.
9. Cartwright A. *Human relations and hospital care.* London: Routledge and Kegan Paul, 1964.
10. Cartwright A, Anderson R. *General practice revisited.* London: Tavistock, 1981.
11. Dixon P, Carr-Hill R. *The NHS and its customers.* III: *Customer feedback surveys—a review of current practice.* York: Centre for Health Economics, University of York, 1989.
12. Department of Health and Social Security. *NHS management enquiry* (Chairman R. Griffiths). London: HMSO, 1983.
13. Secretary of State for Health. *Working for patients.* London: HMSO, 1989.
14. Murray J. A follow-up comparison of patient satisfaction among pre-paid and fee-for-service patients. *Journal of Family Practice* 1988; **26:** 576–81.
15. Deyo R, Diehl A, Rosenthal M. How many days of bed rest for acute back pain? A randomized clinical trial. *New England Journal of Medicine* 1986; **315:** 1064–70.
16. Davies A, Ware J, Brook R, *et al.* Consumer acceptance of prepaid and fee-for-service medical care: results from a randomized controlled trial. *Health Services Research* 1986; **21:** 430–52.
17. Davies A, Ware J. Involving consumers in quality of care assessment. *Health Affairs* 1988; **7:** 3–48.
18. Bradley C, Lewis K. Measures of psychological well-being and treat-

ment satisfaction developed from the responses of people with tablet treated diabetes. *Diabetic Medicine* 1990; **7:** 445–51.

19. Fitzpatrick R, Bury M, Frank A, Donnelly T. Problems in the assessment of outcome in a back pain clinic. *International Rehabilitation Studies* 1987; **9:** 161–5.

20. Blanchard C, Labrecque M, Ruckdeschel J, Blanchard E. Physician behaviors, patient perceptions, and patient characteristics as predictors of satisfaction of hospitalized adult cancer patients. *Cancer* 1990; **65:** 186–92.

21. Romm F, Hulka B, Mayo F. Correlates of outcomes in patients with congestive heart failure. *Medical Care* 1976; **14:** 765–76.

22. Balsdon M, Charlton B, Curran B, Singha H. A survey of attitudes of patients in a department of genito-urinary medicine. *British Journal of Venereology* 1978; **54:** 199–200.

23. Korsch B, Gozzi E, Francis V. Gaps in doctor–patient communications. I: Doctor–patient interaction and patient satisfaction. *Pediatrics* 1968; **42 :**855–71.

24. Savage R, Armstrong D. Effect of general practitioners' consulting style on patients' satisfaction: a controlled study. *British Medical Journal* 1990; **301:** 968–70.

25. Fitzpatrick R. Surveys of patient satisfaction. I: Important general considerations. *British Medical Journal* 1991; **302:** 887–9.

26. McIver S. *Obtaining views of users of health services.* London: King's Fund Centre for Health Services Development, 1991.

27. Feinstein A. Clinical biostatistics. XLI. Hard science, soft data and the challenges of choosing clinical variables in research. *Clinical Pharmacology and Therapeutics* 1977; **22:** 485–98.

28. Fitzpatrick R, Hopkins A. Patients' satisfaction with communication in neurological outpatient clinics. *Journal of Psychosomatic Research* 1981; **25:** 329–34.

29. Kincey J, Bradshaw P, Ley P. Patients' satisfaction and reported acceptance of advice in general practice. *Journal of the Royal College of General Practitioners* 1975; **25:** 558–66.

30. Ley P, Whitworth M, Skilbeck C, Woodward R, Pinsent R, Pike L, *et al.* Improving doctor–patient communications in general practice. *Journal of the Royal College of General Practitioners* 1976; **26:** 720–4.

31. Roghmann K, Hengst A, Zastowny T. Satisfaction with medical care: its measurement and relation to utilisation. *Medical Care* 1979; **17:** 461–77.

32. Orton M, Fitzpatrick R, Fuller A, Mant D, Mlynek C, Thorogood M. Factors affecting women's response to an invitation to attend for a second breast cancer screening examination. *British Journal of General Practice* 1991;**41:**320–3.

33. Weiss B, Senf J. Patient satisfaction survey instrument for use in health maintenance organisations. *Medical Care* 1990; **28:** 434–45.

34. Baker R, Whitfield M. Measuring patient satisfaction: a test of construct validity. *Quality in Health Care* 1992; **1:** 104–9.

35. Pryn J, Rijckman R, van Brunschot C, van den Borne H. Cancer patients' personality characteristics, physician–patient communication and adoption of the Moerman diet. *Social Science and Medicine* 1985: **20:** 831–47.

36. Fitzpatrick R, Hopkins A, Harvard-Watts O. Social dimensions of healing: a longitudinal study of outcomes of medical management of headaches. *Social Science and Medicine* 1983; **17:** 501–10.

37. Hall J, Feldstein M, Fretwell M, *et al.* Older patients' health status and satisfaction with medical care in an HMO population. *Medical Care* 1990; **28:** 261–70.

38. Deyo R, Diehl A. Patient satisfaction with medical care for low back pain. *Spine* 1986; **11:** 28–30.

39. Headache Study Group of University of Western Ontario. Predictors of outcome in headache patients presenting to family physicians. *Headache* 1986; **26:** 285–94.

40. Wooley F, Kane R, Hughes C. The effects of doctor–patient communication on satisfaction and outcome of care. *Social Science and Medicine* 1978; **12:** 123–8.

41. Patrick D, Scrivens E, Charlton J. Disability and patient satisfaction with medical care. *Medical Care* 1983; **21:** 1062–75.

42. Linn L, Greenfield S. Patient suffering and patient satisfaction among the chronically ill. *Medical Care* 1982; **20:** 425–31.

43. Cleary P, Edgman-Levitan S, Roberts M, Moloney T, McMullen W, Walker J, *et al.* Patients evaluate their hospital care: a national survey. *Health Affairs* 1991; **10:** 254–67.

44. Greenley J, Young T, Schoenherr R. Psychological distress and patient satisfaction. *Medical Care* 1982; **20:** 373–85.

45. Williams S, Calnan M. Key determinants of consumer satisfaction with general practice. *Family Practice* 1991; **8:** 237–42.

46. DiMatteo M, Taranta A, Friedman H, Prince L. Predicting patient satisfaction from physicians' non-verbal communication skills. *Medical Care* 1980; **18;** 376–87.

47. Stiles W, Putnam S, Wolf M, James S. Interaction exchange structure and patient satisfaction with medical interviews. *Medical Care* 1979; **17:** 667–81.

48. Roter D. Which facets of communication have strong effects on outcome: a meta-analysis. In: Stewart M, Roter D, eds. *Communicating with medical patients.* London: Sage, 1989.

49. Pendleton D. Doctor–patient communication: a review. In: Pendleton D, Hasler J, eds. *Doctor–patient communication.* London: Academic Press, 1983.

50. Howe J, Porter M, Heaney D, Hopton J. Long to short consultation ratio: a proxy measure of quality of care for general practice. *British Journal of General Practice* 1991; **41:** 48–54.

51. Hjortdahl P, Laerum E. Continuity of care in general practice: effect on patient satisfaction. *British Medical Journal* 1992; **304:** 1287–90.

52. Stewart M, Roter D, eds. *Communicating with medical patients.* London: Sage, 1989.

53. Hall J, Dornan M. What patients think about their medical care and how often they are asked: a meta-analysis of the satisfaction literature. *Social Science and Medicine* 1988; **27:** 935–9.

54. Sira ZB. Affective and instrumental components in the physician–patient relationship. *Journal of Health and Social Behavior* 1980; **21:** 170–80.

55. Ware J, Snyder M. Dimensions of patient attitudes regarding doctors and medical care services. *Medical Care* 1975; **13:** 669–79.
56. Fitzpatrick R, Hopkins A. Problems in the conceptual framework of patient satisfaction research. *Sociology of Health and Illness* 1983; **5:** 297–311.
57. Baker R. Development of a questionnaire to assess patients' satisfaction with consultations in general practice. *British Journal of General Practice* 1990; **40:** 487–90.
58. Nguyen T, Attkisson C, Stegner B. Assessment of patient satisfaction: development and refinement of a service evaluation questionnaire. *Evaluation and Program Planning* 1983; **6:** 299–314.
59. Cox D, Fitzpatrick R, Fletcher A, Gore S, Jones D, Spiegelhalter D. Quality of life assessment: can we keep it simple? *Journal of the Royal Statistical Society* 1992; **A155:** 353–93.
60. Moores B, Thompson A. An all consuming view. *Health Service Journal* 1986; 4 Aug: 880–1.
61. Ware J, Hays R. Methods for measuring patient satisfaction with specific medical encounters. *Medical Care* 1988; **26:** 393–402.
62. Oppenheim A. *Questionnaire design and attitude measurement.* London: Heinemann, 1966.
63. Aaronson N. Quality of life assessment in clinical trials: methodological issues. *Controlled Clinical Trials* 1989; **10:** 195S–208S.
64. Martin E. Consumer evaluation of human services. *Social Policy and Administration* 1986; **20:** 185–200.
65. Linn L, DiMatteo R, Cope D, Robbins A. Measuring physicians' humanistic attitudes, values and behaviors. *Medical Care* 1987; **25:** 504–15.
66. Roter D, Hall J, Katz N. Relations between physicians; behaviors and analogue patients' satisfaction, recall and impressions. *Medical Care* 1987; **25:** 437–51.
67. Fitzpatrick R. Surveys of patient satisfaction. II: Designing a questionnaire and conducting a survey. *British Medical Journal* 1991;**302:** 1129–32.
68. Raftery J, Zarb G. Satisfaction guaranteed? *Health Service Journal* 1990; **100:** 1692–3.

# 2 | Inpatients' opinions of the quality of acute hospital care: discrimination as the key to measurement validity

**Andrew Thompson**
*Cardiff Business School*

Interest in patients' opinions of the quality of hospital care has been growing apace. However, while research on patient satisfaction has been underway for some 35 years, it is only relatively recently that interest has been shown by practitioners and managers of health services. In Britain much impetus was given to the establishment of quality assurance in the National Health Service (NHS) by the Griffiths report which laid special emphasis on the need to seek out the views of those on the receiving end of services.[1]

This new-found focus of attention on 'consumerism' in the NHS has been brought about by quite disparate ideological pressures,[2] as well as being conditioned by what its protagonists intend to use it for within the framework of public services.[3] However, it was clear until the late 1970s that the extant measurement tools did not provide managers or practitioners with information that was action-focused. Either the data, usually generated by surveys, lacked sufficient detail, or it effectively swamped the manager by failing to provide a key to its analysis. While there are many explanations for the failure of services to respond to public concerns, these criticisms of measurement are in part responsible and provide the framework for the research outlined here.

Measurement allows the evaluation of services to take place against standards of good practice, in a way that provides accountability to the public and drives forward the pursuit of improvement in quality by the providers of services. Measurement is integral to the monitoring process of audit and to the regulation of service delivery. Measurement provides a means of establishing the magnitude of an issue in absolute terms, as well as permitting comparisons in relative terms. Therefore the key criterion is that a measurement tool must be able to discriminate between different manifestations of a service, whether it is to compare groups or institutions, or to show changes over time. What issues to measure and how to collect the data are important related concerns, although the latter is beyond the scope of this discussion.

## Methodological issues in questionnaire design

### Content

The philosophy of the approach adopted here is rooted in the belief that, if the views of hospital inpatients are to be reflected in a meaningful way, the patients themselves must determine what issues are pertinent to their care. Furthermore, it is considered to be of critical importance that attention be paid to the means of articulating such views. Hence, an ethnographic methodology has been employed in the development stage, through unstructured and semi-structured interviews in the homes of patients discharged from hospital, in order to allow patients to 'set the agenda' and to do so in their 'natural' language. This approach has been discussed elsewhere in various contexts of health care delivery, including acute inpatients,[4] outpatients[5] and maternity services.[6] A similar initial approach is described in Chapter 5. In essence, this approach allows a qualitative exploration and recording of people's feelings and opinions as they wish to articulate them, using tape recorders and interviewer completed notes, sometimes supplemented by respondent completed diaries. This permits the researcher to understand the matters that concern people, and to learn how widely their views range on each issue. In turn this provides the building material for the development of more structured forms of questioning, as well as helping to interpret quantitative data. It therefore contributes to both content and explanation in surveys of public opinion.

### Form of questions

One of the major problems which has been highlighted in previous research is the lack of clearly distinguishable outcomes between groups of patients. For example, the King's Fund questionnaire, developed by Raphael,[7] produced extremely high proportions of respondents who expressed satisfaction with care, ranging from 93% to 100% in her initial study. Clearly it is impossible to compare wards or hospitals in any meaningful way with these results, since what difference is there between perfection and 7% less than perfection? Besides the problem of poor question design, the alternative explanation would probably be sampling error in this instance.

The phenomenon of apparently high levels of satisfaction is a common finding in this type of research.[8] Does this mean that the public is generally satisfied with the quality of care in acute hospitals? Even if it does, can it be said that this satisfaction extends to every component of care? This latter point seems less tenable, given the presence of complaints, particularly over aspects of communication. Although many people do not complain because they do not know how to do so, or more significantly do not believe that anything would change as a result,[9] there were still more than 30,000 written complaints in England and Wales in 1988/89.[10] Locker and Dunt have argued that questions that embody aggregation of views tend to bias measures towards the positive end of the scale.[11] One reason for this kind of finding may be the lack of specificity in the questions. If answers were required to questions that were highly specific in detail and sensitive to individuals' actual experiences, this would most likely lead to differences between patients' perceptions being revealed. It would then be possible to compare wards, specialties, or any patient group of interest, by appropriate aggregation. This is what provides the focus which will be explored in this chapter, namely the development of measures sufficiently specific and sensitive to discriminate between different experiences of care.

The key to measurement must be in the discriminating ability of the measuring instrument, since any tool that cannot detect actual differences is valueless and fails as an information device.

The development of discriminating measures is an extremely time-consuming activity, and the process took more than 2 years for the acute inpatient questionnaire I developed in the late 1970s.[4] The objective was to spread the respondents across the range of possible answers in an optimal way. Optimality here refers to a combination of qualitative meaning and sufficient support in the population, such that scales do not present an unrealistic number of options or ones that do not secure adequate response.

An example of this process is demonstrated with regard to the issue of arrival at the ward when first admitted to hospital (Table 1). The general format is akin to presenting a statement with which a respondent may strongly agree, or agree, or disagree, or strongly disagree. While this Likert style method offers a clear ordinal scale, it is felt that a more 'naturalistic' approach is to flesh out what each of these responses would mean to a member of the public. Hence, a strongly positive statement is offered at one end of the scale, down to a strongly negative statement at the other. However, given the actual distribution of opinions, it is likely that the

**Table 1.** Example of development of questions.

| | % |
|---|---|
| *Phase 1* | |
| Having arrived at the ward, I found that: | |
|   I quickly adapted to the new routine | 64 |
|   It took me quite a while to condition myself to it | 22 |
|   It took me some little time to fully comprehend what was going on around me | 11 |
|   I was utterly confused | 3 |
| *Phase 2* | |
| Having arrived at the ward, I found that: | |
|   I was able to adapt quickly to the new routine | 44 |
|   It didn't take me long to get accustomed to it | 43 |
|   It took me quite a while to get used to the new routine | 7 |
|   I was confused for quite some time as to what was going on around me | 6 |
| *Phase 3* | |
| Having arrived at the ward, I found that: | |
|   I was able to adapt quickly to the new way of life | 42 |
|   It didn't take me long to get accustomed to the ward life | 48 |
|   I was confused for quite some time as to what was going on around me | 11 |

resulting shape will be highly skewed. Figure 1 illustrates the distribution for successive versions of the question given in Table 1. Each modification involves an adjustment in the wording to ensure that the respondents are spread out, ideally to represent more closely a normal distribution.

This technique can also be used for developing scales in situations where response patterns are symmetrical but highly leptokurtic in

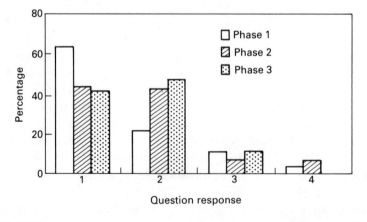

**Fig. 1.** *Distribution of responses on arrival at the ward to different versions of a question; see Table 1.*

shape. This 'peakedness' can be reduced, without removing the symmetry, by offering more choice in the middle of the scale.

The rationale behind this manipulation of the underlying scales is twofold. First, the differences between hospitals, wards or any other groups of patients are often marginal and the subtleties need to be pulled apart in this manner to enable differences to be revealed. This lies at the heart of the discriminating potential of the questions. The second reason for aiming at a more symmetrical distribution concerns the ultimate analysis that is intended. Since this was seen as utilising the statistical theory based on the general linear model, a Gaussian distribution was regarded as the most appropriate.

A further criticism can be levelled at patient satisfaction research that emphasises the derivation of global measures of hospital performance. This is an alluring approach as it attempts to end up with a unitary index that shows whether a particular hospital is good, bad or somewhere in between, in satisfaction terms. A universal indicator has obvious benefits, rather like the economist's focus on money or utility as a baseline standard, but it is highly questionable in the context of patient satisfaction. Even if such a concept could be realised, it would have negligible informational use for developing a hospital's quality assurance programme.

Several studies have attempted to accomplish this for some broad aspects of care, such as nursing care, medical care, food etc.[12] It may be useful to know that the quality of food is unacceptable, but this does not enable management to act unless they know whether the problem lies in the choice, presentation, temperature, or some other component of the food. A problem which may be arguably more serious than the limited utility of global indicators is the possibility that they may mislead managers and practitioners, since global measures are, by definition, aggregates of a variety of experiences.

It follows that what is required is a set of highly specific questions that relate to actual experiences in a way that is sensitive to the nuances of variations in care that result from different contexts. In addition, responses elicited must reflect the differences between individuals' perceptions of a common event. The process of determining the issues and the language to be employed in surveys, discussed above, is a way of ensuring that a patient questionnaire reflects the patients' agenda.

While it makes sense to itemise the components of quality, the converse problem of overwhelming managers and practitioners with voluminous data may arise. The pertinent issues may be in there somewhere, but exactly where and with what importance remains unclear. The key message here is that data, whether collected by survey or not, do not constitute information unless they answer certain questions or provide direction for action. What is required therefore is a key to analysing the data that focuses attention on the pertinent matters in a way that enables priorities to be established.

Conceptually, the hypothesis being put forward here, and by Ray Fitzpatrick in Chapter 1, is that quality is perceived as a multi-dimensional construct, and the resultant expression of satisfaction or dissatisfaction relates to these dimensions. The task of the research is to determine what these dimensions are.

*Form of questionnaire*

The current version of the 'What the patient thinks' acute in-patient questionnaire, last revised in January 1991, contains some 280 items for self-completion by recently discharged patients. The 45 pages are presented in large type to facilitate completion by those with impaired vision, as well as to avoid an appearance of density of questions. There are multicoloured sections to stimulate completion and to allow respondents to tackle just one section if they so desire. A number of design features have been incorporated to minimise the negative effect of questionnaire length. In addition, the survey is managed and administered by a national charity, the Health Policy Advisory Unit, which has the advantage of being seen to be independent and publicly accountable.

The format of the questionnaire leads respondents through a logical progression from pre-admission, including previous experience and prior information, through admission and the residential phase, including physical aspects, interpersonal relationships, information and communication, to discharge arrangements and after-care. A few summary questions are included to allow insight into how generalised views are formed, as well as to derive the priorities referred to earlier.

## Analysis and results

The identification of dimensions of satisfaction and dissatisfaction was carried out through the statistical technique of factor analysis, by identifying clusters of individual aspects that are strongly associated in both a statistical and a substantive sense. The original analysis was based on a survey of 1,357 patients across seven hospitals within

**Table 2.** Dimensions of perceptions of quality of care.

| Dimension | Number of questions | Common variance |
|---|---|---|
| Medical care and information | 25 | 51% |
| Food and physical facilities | 16 | 15% |
| Ward atmosphere | 16 | 9% |
| Nursing care | 16 | 8% |
| Quantity of food | 4 | 6% |
| Visiting arrangements | 4 | 6% |

five English Regions.[4] Six dimensions of patients' perceptions of care were identified using factor analysis and employing varimax orthogonal rotation to maximise the variance that is explained for each question in any one factor.[13] The final selection of questions to be included in this analysis was confined to the 71 that met a number of statistical and psychometric criteria. These included a Kaiser–Meyer–Olkin measure of sampling adequacy[14] of 0.89, communalities of between 0.165 and 0.669, factor loadings that demonstrated substantive as well as statistically significant levels, and factors that were intuitively meaningful and independent of each other.

The dimensions shown in Table 2 comprise varying numbers of questions, based on the responses of between 479 and 1,093 patients, and are ordered to reflect the amount of explanation of common variance. A few questions appear on more than one factor owing to their complexity, although this is kept to a minimum. The remaining variance is explained by a seventh independent factor which emerged relating to perceptions of staff workload rather than quality of care *per se.*

By way of illustration, Table 3 lists, in order of factor loading (ie a measure of the amount of question variance in common with the other questions in the same factor), the questions that comprise the dimension relating to medical care and information. This label, applied after inspection of these variables, implies that patients perceive information to be related to the doctors' responsibilities, irrespective of the source and of how well that responsibility is executed.

Underlying dimensions such as these empirically derived ones are a useful basis for simplifying a complex mix of questions typically generated for use in a survey. However, while they can be used to focus attention on the broader issues for consideration and ultimately action, there is no indication of the relative importance

**Table 3.** Dimension relating to medical care and information.

| Question topic | Factor loading |
| --- | --- |
| Prompting of information from doctors | 0.80 |
| Prompting of information from nurses | 0.69 |
| Explanation of information by doctors | 0.68 |
| Prompting of information from paramedicals | 0.65 |
| Amount of information from doctors | 0.64 |
| Method of explanation by doctors | 0.54 |
| Confidence in doctors | 0.52 |
| Duration of doctors' visits | 0.49 |
| Overall care by doctors | 0.49 |
| Amount of information from nurses | 0.47 |
| After-care from outpatient department | 0.41 |
| Explanation of information by paramedicals | 0.41 |
| Overall personal care in hospital | 0.40 |
| Frequency of doctors' visits | 0.39 |
| Reliability of information from staff | 0.39 |
| Ease of understanding staff | 0.38 |
| Confidence in paramedicals | 0.38 |
| First reaction on arrival at hospital | 0.32 |
| Amount of information from visitors | 0.31 |
| Organisation of ward routine | 0.31 |
| Care on leaving hospital | 0.30 |
| Care on admission to hospital | 0.30 |
| Privacy during doctors' examinations | 0.28 |
| Explanation of information by nurses | 0.27 |
| Boredom | 0.24 |

that should be attached to each dimension. As a method of deriving patient-centred care, it follows that not only should the public be listened to for establishing the domain of concerns but also they should indicate the relative weight to be given to the components of care. Patient-determined priorities for both the positive and negative aspects of hospital care can be established to accomplish this weighting procedure.

The national database now includes the results from surveys in more than 100 acute hospitals across Britain, involving more than 80,000 patients over 14 years. A sample of 20 hospitals surveyed during 1987–1990, prior to major revisions in the questionnaire, illustrates the way in which priorities become established. Table 4

**Table 4.** Best aspects of care in hospital.

| Rank | Aspect of care | Weight |
| --- | --- | --- |
| 1 | Nursing care | 23% |
| 2 | Doctors' care | 18% |
| 3 | Cleanliness | 7% |
| 4 | Relationships with staff | 7% |
| 5 | Relationships with other patients | 5% |
| 6 | Paramedical care | 5% |
| 7 | Nursing auxiliaries'/domestics' care | 5% |

shows the aspects of care that attract at least 5% of the total weight, as a proportion of the total given for the 23 aspects offered for selection, on which detailed questions have already been answered. With the exception of cleanliness, these aspects are concerned with the *content* of care, with a focus on interpersonal relationships in hospital.

Table 5 shows those aspects of care in need of most improvement. They are more concerned with the *context* of care.

Although the national weightings will vary over time, the increasing size of the database will lead to a large degree of stability. From an individual hospital point of view, there can be much to learn from comparisons with these national data, which may reveal differently ranked aspects, or variations in weighting.

As an aid to the management of services, what is proposed here is a combination of both the statistical and patient-determined approaches, to enable focus to be given to the most important aspects of service delivery, both in a positive mode of reinforcing good practice and in a corrective mode of improving the quality of

**Table 5.** Aspects in need of most improvement.

| Rank | Aspect of care | Weight |
| --- | --- | --- |
| 1 | Food | 14% |
| 2 | Things to do in the ward | 13% |
| 3 | Information | 7% |
| 4 | Temperature | 6% |
| 5 | Facilities on the ward | 6% |
| 6 | Sleep | 6% |
| 7 | Level of noise | 6% |
| 8 | Decor | 6% |

**Table 6.** Satisfaction with medical care.

|  | UK (%) | A (%) | Z (%) |
|---|---|---|---|
| (i) The doctors' visits were few and far between/extremely rare | 20 | 12 | 28 |
| (ii) The doctors were remarkably friendly and sociable at all times | 57 | 76 | 14 |
| (iii) I had absolute confidence in everything the doctors did for me | 54 | 63 | 12 |

delivery. Attention needs to be given both to aspects that satisfy and those that dissatisfy if quality is to be assured from the public perspective. A specific example of this approach in the context of oncology hospital care has been explained elsewhere.[15]

In order to illustrate how well individual questions can discriminate between hospitals, and by implication between wards, specialties and any other grouping of interest, some topics have been chosen from the dimension relating to medical care and information. The data have been selected from the same sample as that shown with reference to the patient-determined priorities. The results in Table 6 show the national average score (UK) alongside the highest (A) and lowest (Z) ratings found in the sample. In an attempt to demonstrate this in the most lucid way, only statements from one extreme of a particular question are presented, either positive or negative in orientation. The ratings of doctors in the UK are seen to be generally high, but while some hospitals such as A score extremely highly there are also worryingly low scores. Absolute confidence may seem a little foolhardy, but it is extremely disturbing to note how low hospital Z was rated, particularly bearing in mind that this is an average score for that hospital, suggesting even lower scores for certain wards.

Information and communication clearly affect the whole process of hospital care, from pre-admission to post-discharge, as illustrated in Table 7. The provision of information prior to a period of stay can help in preparing someone for what may be a confusing and worrying episode. This is also important to enable people to make domestic arrangements as necessary, particularly where dependants are involved. Patients often need to prompt staff into giving information, if they have the courage to ask. For example, more than a quarter found this was necessary with the doctors, and the proportion was nearly a half in one hospital. Even a demand for information does not guarantee that sufficient will be given. Overall, about one in seven patients felt that both nurses and doctors left them seriously underinformed, although this varied between one in twenty and one in four. Not only the quantity is

**Table 7.** Satisfaction with information.

|  | UK (%) | A (%) | Z (%) |
|---|---|---|---|
| (i) I always had to demand/it was often necessary to ask for information about my treatment from the doctors | 27 | 17 | 44 |
| (ii) There were a lot of undesirable gaps in the information from the: Nurses | 13 | 4 | 24 |
| Doctors | 15 | 6 | 24 |
| (iii) Whenever the doctors had any instructions or information for me they always discussed it with me | 67 | 89 | 55 |
| (iv) At no time did I feel that the truth about my condition was being hidden from me | 88 | 91 | 79 |
| (v) I got the impression that the staff were not always sure about the information they gave me | 18 | 9 | 21 |
| (vi) I had to ask for advice about what I should or should not do after leaving hospital | 34 | 23 | 50 |
| (vii) On leaving hospital I was given no advice at all | 17 | 11 | 22 |

important, but also the method of communicating information. Where patients feel that they are participating in the process, rather than on the receiving end, they are more likely to respond positively to information giving. The use of a third party to convey information may be a sound policy, but it has to be seen as such by the recipient to avoid a feeling of low status in the transaction.

Doubts relating to the perceived truth or reliability of the information provided can lead to breakdowns in trust between patient and carer. In general, these do not appear to reveal any major problems, although more than a fifth of patients in one hospital are not assured on these issues.

The importance of the discharge phase needs to be emphasised, especially concerning the provision of information about after-care and follow-up treatment where necessary. The period of notice, informing of friends and relatives, and advice about what to do, or not do, are components of this. It is somewhat disconcerting that at least a quarter, and in one case half, of discharged patients had to prompt for advice. Even so, a large number still felt that they were given no advice at all. One of the possible problems here is that they may have forgotten or not understood information given at this stage. However, if subsequently they do not remember it, this raises a problem that needs solving if certain rehabilitative behaviour is to be adhered to. The provision of written as well as orally communicated material, plus the reinforcement by all relevant staff, from hospital to community, can help to resolve this.

Crude comparisons between hospitals are dangerous insofar as often there are differences in resources, casemix and other factors, which can mean that like is not compared with like. This would be fair comment if the responses were to assume, without further investigation, that an 'A' score was good and a 'Z' score bad, but the measurement issue still stands up if these different contexts can be shown to produce different perceptions among their users. In other words, different experiences of care are likely to result from different ways of providing services, and a valid measurement tool must be able to show these in a meaningful way. It is believed that this is an essential, although not sufficient, condition for claiming validity in measurement. Other concerns include such issues as content validity, discussed earlier under the agenda setting phase of development, and construct validity (see page 72).

Some of my other publications illustrate the findings for different aspects of care, showing how well scales have been able to reveal differences at the hospital level for both the content and the context of care.[16-20]

The issue of global views of satisfaction with hospital care can now be considered in relation to these more detailed findings. It might be postulated that the crucial question is whether, as a result of one particular experience of hospital care, a patient would consider returning for further treatment, should it prove necessary and given a real choice. The national data show that about 60% of discharged patients would be happy to return to the same hospital, but this can vary from around 80% down to 40%. At the negative end of the spectrum, consistently around 7% of recently discharged patients would prefer to go somewhere else next time, ranging from only 2% up to 20–25%. As argued elsewhere,[21] such figures can be extremely misleading, unless further information is sought for an explanation. The reasons for the response to this question can be most closely identified with aspects of nursing care, medical care and information, and food and physical environment. Even when put together, these three factors still account for only about a quarter of the variation. The response to this question is clearly more complex than we can adequately explain at present.

## Conclusion

The success of any patient survey can probably be gauged in terms of how representative it is in reflecting the views of the population who use hospitals, and to what extent it leads to continuous quality improvement in service delivery. The response rate that is currently achieved with the questionnaires that I have developed is close to 70%, although lower returns are a feature of inner-city areas, especially in London. This is probably due to a number of factors, including mobility, deprivation, homelessness etc. This response rate compares favourably with many postal surveys, despite concerns about the length of the questionnaire. Part of the explanation for such a good response rate is likely to be that the topic itself is viewed as being important by the general public, especially given the public's allegiance to the NHS as an institution. Another factor is believed to be the degree of sensitivity of the issues raised and the specificity of the question wording to people's personal experiences. The more generalised a set of questions the less likely it is to evoke a response. Since the questions, and associated wording were derived from the public in the first place, it is no surprise that the questionnaire is seen as relevant and insightful.

It is argued here that if information on the quality of inpatient hospital care is to be obtained, measures are required that can distinguish between the different experiences in a way that indicates areas and priorities for action. It is believed that this can only be accomplished through highly specific and sensitive questions, which then need to be composited and weighted to transform data into information. Only when this happens will we be in a position to see more clearly and in a more comprehensive way what patients actually think. The onus is then on managers and practitioners to assure a high quality of service to all patients.

## References

1. Department of Health and Social Security. *NHS management enquiry* (Chairman: R. Griffiths). London: HMSO, 1983.
2. Thompson AGH. The practical implications of patient satisfaction research. *Health Services Management Research.* 1988; 1(2):112–9.
3. Pfeffer N, Coote A. *Is quality good for you?* Social Policy Paper No. 5. London: Institute for Public Policy Research, 1991.
4. Thompson AGH. *The measurement of patients' perceptions of the quality of hospital care.* Unpublished doctoral thesis, University of Manchester, 1983.
5. Thompson AGH. *The outpatients' agenda.* Paper at 7th Conference of the International Society of Quality Assurance in Health Care, Stockholm, Sweden, 1990.
6. Thompson AGH, Whelan A. *Assessing women's perceptions of obstetrical care: a qualitative research agenda.* Paper presented at the 1st International Conference on Primary Care Obstetrics and Perinatal Health, 's Hertogenbosch, Netherlands, 1991.

7. Raphael W. *Patients and their hospitals: a survey of patients' views of life in general hospitals.* London: King Edward's Hospital Fund, 1969.
8. Fitzpatrick R. Surveys of patient satisfaction. I. Important general considerations. *British Medical Journal* 1991; **302**: 887–9.
9. Prescott-Clarke P, Brooks T, Machray C. *Focus on health care: surveying the public in four health districts.* London: RIPA/SCPR, 1988.
10. Department of Health. *Return of written complaints by or on behalf of patients: England and Wales, financial year 1988/89.* London: Statistics and Management Information Division, Government Statistical Service, 1990.
11. Locker D, Dunt D. Theoretical and methodological issues in sociological studies of consumer satisfaction with medical care. *Social Science and Medicine* 1978; **12A**:283–92.
12. Kerruish A, Wickings I, Tarrant P. Information from patients as a management tool: empowering managers to improve the quality of care. *Hospital and Health Services Review* 1988; **84**(2): 64–7.
13. Kaiser HF. The varimax criterion for analytic rotation in factor analysis. *Psychometrika* 1958; **23**: 187–200.
14. Kaiser HF, Rice J. Little jiffy, Mark IV. *Educational and Psychological Measurement* 1974; **34**: 111–7.
15. Thompson AGH. What do patients think about specialist cancer centres? In: Pritchard AP, ed. *Cancer nursing: a revolution in care.* London: Macmillan, 1989.
16. Moores B, Thompson AGH. Getting feedback. *Health and Social Service Journal* 1981; **91**: 634–6.
17. Moores B, Thompson AGH. From the patient's mouth. *Health and Social Service Journal* 1985; **95**: 1040–2.
18. Moores B, Thompson AGH. What 1,357 hospital inpatients think about aspects of their stay in British acute hospitals. *Journal of Advanced Nursing* 1986; **11:** 87–102.
19. Moores B, Thompson AGH. An all-consuming view. *Health Service Journal* 1986; **96**: 892–3.
20. Thompson AGH. A patient's eye view. *Nursing Times* 1986; **82**(10): 30–2.
21. Thompson AGH. The soft approach to quality of hospital care. *International Journal of Quality and Reliability Management.* 1986; **3**(3): 57–65.

# 3 | The CASPE patient satisfaction system

**Cathy Gritzner**
*CASPE Research, King Edward's Hospital Fund for London*

Patient satisfaction represents a complex mixture of perceived need, expectations and experience of care. Pascoe defines patient satisfaction as health care recipients' reaction to salient aspects of the context, process and result of their experience.[1]

Interest in measuring patient satisfaction in the National Health Service (NHS) in the UK has been renewed over the past few years. The first reason is the reorganisation of health care which came into effect in April 1991. The NHS now has District Health Authorities (DHAs) and General Practice Fund Holders taking on a new role of purchasing health care services from provider units such as hospitals and community services. There has been much emphasis placed on quality in purchaser contracts. Quality should be an important determinant in the demand for a provider's services. The feedback from patients on their perceptions of the quality of the service received may affect both purchasers' and providers' decisions when subsequent contracts are written. A second reason is that patient satisfaction may be an important prerequisite for high quality care, as it has been shown that satisfied patients are more likely to cooperate effectively with the clinical team and to comply with their recommendations.[2] Third, as highlighted by Williamson, patients have views on virtually everything that is going on, and these frequently differ from those of the professionals caring for them.[3] Information from patient satisfaction surveys can therefore identify patients' differing perspectives, to be considered by medical and clinical audit teams. Finally, reflecting increasing consumerism in society, members of the public demand that they should be given greater choice and information in relation to their care.

Most published work on patient satisfaction considers the satisfaction of patients, with the notable exception of that of Raphael and Mandeville who focused on outpatient services.[4] Early studies include those of McGhee who interviewed 490 adults in different wards in an Edinburgh teaching hospital.[5] Cartwright carried out the first national study using questionnaires covering many aspects of hospital life,[6] whilst Carstairs focused work on communication but gathered some useful information for patients on their hospital care.[7]

Most studies since the 1970s have been carried out at a local rather than a national level. One reason for this is the advent of local Community Health Care Councils (CHCs) in 1974. Most CHC reports have not been published. From a review of academic studies and the CHC reports that are available, Jones *et al* found that the times at which patients are wakened, facilities for washing, bathing, lavatories, noise, smoking arrangements and ward amenities such as day rooms and television have consistently produced the highest level of dissatisfaction for inpatients.[8] For outpatients the dissatisfaction has focused around waiting times and the lack of amenities such as refreshments, reading materials, and facilities for children. Most studies used self-report questionnaires completed by the patient.

It is against this background that CASPE Research has designed a patient satisfaction tool, supported by a grant from the Department of Health. It is designed to measure inpatient and outpatient satisfaction using separate questionnaires, and to provide a management tool for the continuous monitoring of satisfaction. Particular emphasis is placed on continuous monitoring, as a study by Hyde-Pryce showed that one-off surveys tended to be ignored by managers.[9] Research on the CASPE inpatient questionnaire has shown, in contrast, that executive action is more likely to be taken if managers receive patients' views on a regular basis.[10]

There are three alternative CASPE systems that can now be used: a computerised version, a manual version and a stand-alone software model. The most versatile is the computerised version which is linked into the hospital's patient administration system (PAS) or hospital information system (HISS) which provides patients' details such as name, sex, ward or specified clinic. This information is already entered on to the local PAS system in many hospitals, and the number is growing. Figure 1 shows how the CASPE system receives patient detail download from the PAS on to a personal computer (PC), which is used to generate specific questionnaires and personalised letters. Patients are given the letter and questionnaire at the registration desk for outpatients, or in the ward for inpatients. They are requested to put their completed and anonymous questionnaires, and any extra comments that they may wish to make, in sealed boxes located on the wards or in the outpatient areas.

The patients' responses are read by an optical mark reader

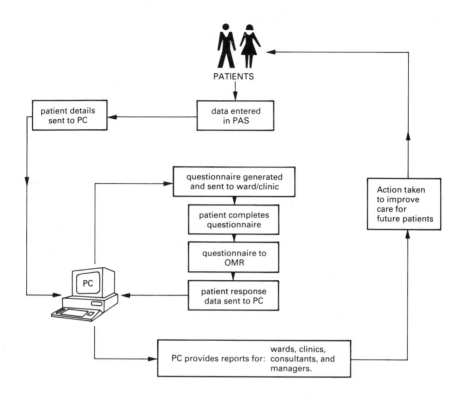

**Fig. 1.** *Computerised CASPE system: flow diagram.*

(OMR) operated centrally by CASPE. Bar coding on the questionnaire allows the data to be summarised by clinic, ward, consultant,
patient's age, or any other field recorded routinely in the PAS. The
aggregated response data are then sent back to the hospital's PC
or main computer system to produce local reports at ward or clinic
level, or more widely, for consultants and managers.

A manual system has also been developed to take account of
those health authorities that do not have certain specialties or outpatient data on their PAS. This means that the completed questionnaire cannot be linked to a patient's recorded administrative
data, and a generalised letter only is given. This limits the reporting facility, and reports can only be aggregated to a distribution
point such as a ward, clinic consultant or specialty.

Stand-alone software has also been written so that questionnaires can be generated for areas where it is not possible or practical to download data or pre-coded questionnaires.

## Questionnaires

The core questionnaires for both inpatients and outpatients contain questions about topics that have been identified by patients as being important to their care. An analysis of several hundred semi-structured interviews in 1987/88 with both inpatients and outpatients in Bloomsbury provided a list of topics and words that patients used to discuss services. These were ranked and selected for inclusion in the relevant questionnaire. The core questionnaires therefore reflect issues that are important to patients rather than reflecting areas of concern to staff. The topics covered by both the inpatient and outpatient questionnaires incorporate clinical treatment, hotel services, ward facilities and organisational aspects of care.

One page of the inpatient questionnaire is shown in Fig. 2. Patients are asked to fill in the box that most reflects their perception of that particular topic. The scaling of very satisfied, satisfied, somewhat dissatisfied, very dissatisfied is based on a four-point Likert scale. The CASPE questionnaire also includes, on the reverse, up to thirteen additional topics with questions generated by local managers and clinicians, such as satisfaction with policies about smoking and about privacy. Examples of additional features on the outpatient questionnaire include the presence of medical students during consultation and the use of pharmacy facilities.

Managers need to know the precise reason for dissatisfaction amongst patients. If managers cannot identify from the aggregated data the cause of any problem, a series of second level questionnaires is available for a deeper analysis of any particular area. These questionnaires are intended to provide a detailed 'snapshot' of a service. Subsidiary questionnaires relating to noise, bathrooms and lavatories, food, pain control, and the organisation of wards are available. We have also developed a questionnaire relating to doctors, and are working on one for nurses. There are also questionnaires specific for the different services offered in hospitals. So far these include obstetrics, antenatal care, acute psychiatry, accident and emergency, genito-urinary medicine, paediatrics and intensive care.

In more than 700 interviews with patients, Smith found that 86% of respondents experienced no problems in understanding the content of the CASPE questionnaires. However, five questions, relating to the organisation of the ward, 'atmosphere', clinical treatment, nurses, doctors and ward surroundings, proved to be

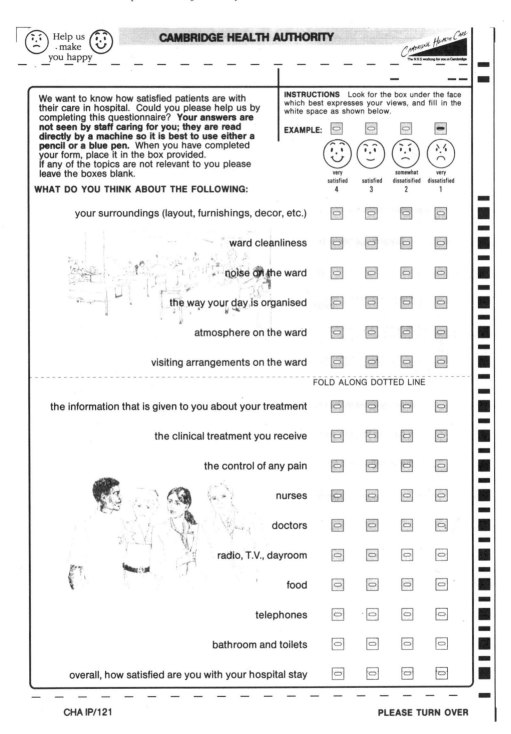

**Fig. 2.** *One side of the inpatient questionnaire sheet.*

worded unsuccessfully and have been changed.[11] This study also confirmed the generally high levels of satisfaction recorded by inpatients, especially in regard to their nursing and medical staff. The questionnaires also revealed measurable differences in patient satisfaction between hospitals.

The CASPE system was installed in seven research districts providing a reasonable cross-section of sizes and types of DHA in the NHS. The CASPE system is now also being used commercially by more than 20 Health Authorities and Disablement Service Centres. Clients receive advice on the introduction of the system and are trained in the use of the software. Experience gained in the research sites has enabled CASPE to help providers establish the patient satisfaction system so that staff training can now be completed and printing and distribution of questionnaires begun within 3 months of acceptance of the quotation.

## Response rates

Response rates have varied between the six research Health Authorities. It has not proved possible to obtain a response from every patient owing to organisational factors within the hospitals. Problems include delays in the internal post and the movement of patients between wards. In order to increase response rates and gain greater patient participation, there have been various initiatives. The core questionnaires, for both inpatients and outpatients, have been translated into Polish, Bengali, Chinese, Turkish, French and German. Interpreters have been used in two DHAs to help pregnant Bengali women who cannot read or write to complete the questionnaires. Volunteers have been used in outpatient eye clinics to help elderly patients or those who have had eye drops inserted. Questionnaires are also available in Braille, Moon and large-print versions.

## Additional comments

Apart from filling in the questionnaires, patients are also encouraged to give additional written comments. They often take the opportunity to do this, their confidentiality being assured by the system. Some recent outpatient comments are:

> 'The chairs in the corridor are too close; there is no elbow room.'
> 'Timed appointments are a waste of time unless patients are seen on time.'

'Car parking is impossible.'
'Highly professional and I was treated as a human being.'
'Everyone I encountered was helpful.'

Amongst inpatient comments are:

'I sometimes wondered who was in charge.'
'Overall my stay was OK, except for the cockroaches.'
'Telephones were not in order throughout an 8-week stay.'
'It is the opinion of all patients in ward X that the food is inedible and it is an insult to expect us to actually eat the rubbish.'

These comments can be grouped into topic areas and provide valuable insights to clinicians and managers, adding information to the statistical data and complementing routine graphical reports. The information can be fed back to patients, as well as to managers and clinicians, in both quantitative and qualitative form (Fig. 3). Some staff now display patients' comments on wards, as well as the bar charts and other graphs, in order to encourage the completion of future questionnaires.

It is also possible to compare ratings between sites, weighting local scores according to age and sex mix. The large dot in

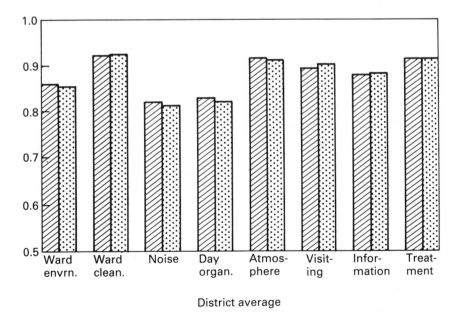

District average

**Fig. 3.** *Inpatient index scores: March 1990.* The eight pairs of columns refer to the score (left) and the district average (right) for the first eight topics on the questionnaire sheet in Fig. 2.

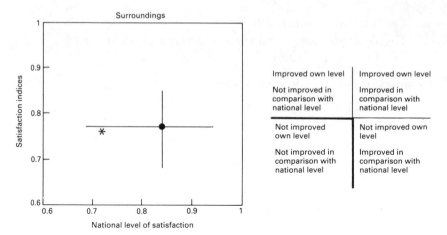

**Fig. 4.** *Patients' perception of ward surroundings.* The large dot indicates the base score for the year, and the star the most recent score.

Fig. 4 represents the previous year's score in two ways: along the horizontal axis it represents the score of all the database sites and along the vertical axis it represents the individual unit's score The star represents the position now. The key is used to interpret the graph. In this example the star is in the bottom left-hand quadrant and indicates that the unit has not improved compared with either its performance last year or the performance of the database sites. This is one way of demonstrating that managerial action should follow to improve the patient satisfaction scores.

We have found that actions taken tend to fall into three categories, requiring no funding, small funds or large funds. However, actions needing no or small funds can result in definite improvements in patient care. For example, a decision that soft-soled shoes would be worn by nursing staff at night followed from low satisfaction scores on the topic of 'noise'. As a second example, when the ward day room was designated as a non-smoking area, levels of satisfaction increased and were maintained.

CASPE surveys have also resulted in the introduction of games for patients to relieve boredom on wards, especially orthopaedic wards, and the provision of more up-to-date toys for children. Hooks have been fixed to doors in washing areas, and toilet areas redesigned for single rather than mixed sex use.

Larger scale projects have included the redesign of waiting and consulting areas in a genito-urinary clinic, in order to give patients more privacy. One hospital's painting programme was also rescheduled to take account of patients' perceptions of the drabness of certain wards.

## Conclusion

The CASPE patient satisfaction system can enable managers in the NHS to know the opinions of their patients and their perceptions of the quality of care. This will become increasingly important as the move towards the internal market and the resulting changes focus purchasers and providers of health care towards the consumer's perspective. Already managers report that hospital staff are more consumer orientated. The CASPE system not only allows the identification of faults but can provide encouragement for further improvement.

## References

1. Pascoe GC. Patient satisfaction on primary health care. *Evaluation and Program Planning* 1983; **6:** 185–210.
2. Donabedian A. *The definition of quality and approaches to its assessment and monitoring.* Vol. 1. Ann Arbor, Michigan: Health Administration Press, 1980.
3. Williamson J. Providing quality care. *Health Services Management* 1991;February: 18–23.
4. Raphael W, Mandeville J. *Being an outpatient.* London: King's Fund, 1977.
5. McGhee A. *The patient's attitude to nursing care.* Edinburgh: Livingstone, 1961.
6. Cartwright A. *Human relations and hospital care.* London: Routledge and Kegan Paul, 1964.
7. Carstairs V. *Channels of communication.* Scottish Health Service Home and Health Department, 1970.
8. Jones L, Leneman L, Maclean U. *Consumer feedback for the NHS.* London: King's Fund, 1987.
9. Hyde-Pryce C. *Our user's voice: the effect of patient opinion surveys on the management of the health service.* 1986. King's Fund College Library. Unpublished.
10. Wickings I. Proof of the pudding. *Health Service Journal* 1989; **99:** 1070–1.
11. Smith C. *A national system for measuring patient satisfaction in the United Kingdom.* Paper presented at the International Society of Quality Assurance in Health Care, 29–31 May 1991.

# 4 | Developing instruments for the measurement of patient satisfaction for Family Health Service Authorities

**Ralph Leavey***
*School of Health, St Martin's College, Lancaster*
**Alison J. Wilson**
*Freelance Research Worker*

There has been increasing pressure on Family Health Service Authorities (FHSAs) to carry out 'satisfaction' surveys of the population registered with general practitioners. The nature and scope of the interactions between health service users and general practitioners are complex. Moreover, FHSAs cover populations that vary by age and socio-economic status, presenting different kinds of needs and demands for services. The potential range of FHSA interest is thus broad, and the concerns of different FHSAs will consequently vary.

Because of this, FHSAs can be faced with bewildering choices when deciding what aspect of satisfaction with services to survey. Decisions about this may be set by national or regional priorities or by FHSA plans or current concerns. Beyond this, FHSAs must still determine precisely what the purpose of the survey is to be, which could include:

- Baseline audit as a first step in planning.
- Identification of unmet need (whether socio-economic, ethnic, geographical or demographic).
- Identification of differences in acceptability of services provided (identifying zones of better practice).
- Evaluation of changes in policy and other interventions (preferably by repeating baseline audits).

Having made the purpose of the survey explicit, the FHSA faces more detailed choices, including:

- What service, and what aspect of that service, to enquire about.
- What population: the whole or part of the FHSA's population or some practice(s), or a sub-group of the population (eg the elderly).

*Formerly Research Fellow, Centre for Primary Care, Department of General Practice, University of Manchester.

- What kinds of information: reported experience; service performance; evaluations of service; wants; express changes required.

Interactions between users and providers are complex. Areas of concern include, for example, accessibility and availability of services, communication, technical quality of care and follow-up. A single 'blanket' questionnaire covering all aspects wastes effort collecting data on aspects about which there is at present little or no concern, or gathers only superficial data about aspects that are a current concern. We have therefore decided in our studies to adopt a modular approach.

The modular design entailed developing a number of instruments, each one focusing on a specific aspect of service delivery. These questionnaire 'modules' would be used alone or in combination. The advantages of such an approach are:

- It provides the capability to go into more detail about specific areas and produce information of greater relevance for service monitoring.
- It gives users of the method more choice over the aspects of the service they choose to investigate: users can survey just one aspect quite cheaply, or can combine several modules.
- It is more cost effective as users can concentrate resources on the aspect they are most keen to survey without having to carry the overhead (in an omnibus survey) of questions in which they have only marginal interest.

This approach also has disadvantages:

- It is more focused: users need to be clearer about their aims at the outset.
- More design work is required to ensure feasible packages if several modules are combined.

Choosing a modular approach means that in the development phase early decisions have to be taken about how many and what aspects of services should be tackled. In our study, this was done both by reviewing previous work and by discussion with end-users (the FHSAs).

Two other constraints were imposed by the FHSAs that commissioned our study: all questionnaires should be designed for self-completion and postal delivery, for reasons of cost; responses should be pre-coded, again for reasons of cost in relation to ease of data entry.

**Development of the questionnaires**

At an early stage discussions were held with collaborating FHSAs. These focused on the balance to be struck between different aspects of services. Lists of possible topics to be included under each heading were discussed and, again, FHSAs were asked to indicate some order of preference. These agreements set out the broad agenda for the project.

The FHSAs that agreed to collaborate with the project team were all in the North Western Health Region and covered a broad spread of settings: Lancashire, Salford, Tameside, and Trafford. Each FHSA agreed to help with pilot work by identifying populations and providing samples. It was also the responsibility of each FHSA to ensure that local representative committees of the contractors (local medical committees and local dental committees) were kept informed about the progress of the project.

Discussions with FHSAs elicited the following order of priority for the development of modules relating to satisfaction with care provided by general practitioners:

(a) Consulting arrangements, waiting times, duration of consultation.
(b) Home and out of hours visiting, telephone contacts, repeat prescribing, results of investigations, certificates, access, surgery premises.
(c) Patient–doctor communication.
(d) Health promotion clinics.
(e) Information for patients.

At the time of writing, 14 modules have been developed and tested. Most of these have been tried in large-scale pilots, and many have also been used in full-scale surveys. A list of the completed modules for general practitioners appears in Table 1.

*Identifying themes and topics for each module*

The framework for many surveys of user opinion of general practitioner services was set by Anne Cartwright almost 25 years ago.[1] Since then there have been other large-scale national surveys which have either repeated or added to the list of topics covered.[2-5] There have also been a number of large regional or multi-locality studies, in South West London,[6] the Manchester area[7,8] and the North West,[9,10] and many studies carried out in particular towns or general practices, ranging in size, scope and quality.

**Table 1.** Completed general practitioner modules.

| Module title | Number of questions | Summary of content |
|---|---|---|
| 1+2. Consulting arrangements | 43 | Hours<br>Appointment systems<br>Queue systems |
| 3. Waiting times | 5 | Length of time before seeing doctor |
| 4. Duration of consultation | 9 | Time spent with general practitioner |
| 5. Home visits | 16 | Requests<br>Wait for visits |
| 6. Out of hours visits | 18 | Requests<br>Wait for visits |
| 7. Repeat prescriptions<br>Investigations<br>Medical certificates | 27 | Systems for obtaining prescriptions etc |
| 8. Telephone advice | 18 | *Ad hoc* consultations<br>Telephone systems |
| 9. Access | 10 | Travel difficulties |
| 10. Premises | 47 | Surgery building<br>Waiting area<br>Privacy |
| 11. Seeing the doctor | 35 | Patient–doctor communication |
| 12. Prevention/promotion | 54 | Health checks<br>Health promotion clinics |
| 13. Information | 25 | Information wanted by user |
| 14. Core/classification | 32 | Use of general practitioner classification |

Previous work was important in three respects: it allowed a long list of topic areas to be drawn up under each of the main themes identified for study; in many cases it helped to put the scale of problems experienced into perspective; it helped to speed up the design process. For some aspects of service delivery, these previous surveys were a major source of both topics and approaches to questioning, so several different variations of a question could be tried in early tests. The main theme(s) of each module were thus derived from reviews of previous work, from discussion with other research workers, and from talking to users. Out of this emerged a more detailed list of topics. For example, in the module focused on patient–doctor contact, the topics included communication, some procedures, advice and knowledge. The module covering consulting arrangements included surgery hours, appointment systems, and the availability of non-urgent and urgent appointments.

The topic list formed the basis for face-to-face open-ended interviews with service users. The aim of these interviews was to ensure that the prospective coverage of the module was adequate and relevant.

### Semi-structured questionnaires

From the open-ended interviews guided by the list of topics, a set of questions was drawn up. The aim was to break down broad topics into questions with a number of possible responses. The semi-structured questionnaires were then tested on quota samples of 30–40 people to check for understanding.

### Structured questionnaires

The results of the semi-structured interviews formed the basis of the first draft of a structured questionnaire. As this was designed for completion by the respondents, the questionnaire had to include instructions about what questions to answer, how to answer, and when to skip questions or sections that were not applicable. Almost all responses were pre-coded in order to ease data entry. These questionnaires were tested in large pilot postal surveys (with samples of between 300 and 600), either singly or in combination with other modules.

The final version of each questionnaire was modified after a review of the results from the pilot work. This might involve the omission or alteration of certain questions and also of the routing instructions, in order to smooth the respondent's passage through the questionnaire. An example from the section on patient–doctor communication is shown in Table 2.

### Combining the modular questionnaires

Final versions of the modules were used in full-scale surveys of FHSA populations. FHSAs wanted to look at several aspects of activity, which meant combining different modules. Whenever several modules were combined, careful thought had to be given to the overall length and layout of the package and the transition from one topic to the next.

**Table 2.** Part of a questionnaire, from the section on patient–doctor communication.

| WHEN YOU SEE YOUR DOCTOR |
| --- |

56.  When you see *your usual* doctor at the surgery how much time does
     he/she spend with you?

     It's usually less than 5 minutes..........................1
     It's usually around about 5 minutes ...............2
     It's usually more than 5 minutes.....................3
     It's usually around 10 minutes.........................4
     It's usually more than 10 minutes...................5
     It's different each time ......................................6

57.  The *last time* you saw *your usual* doctor how much time did he/she
     spend with you?

     Less than 5 minutes.........................................1
     Around about 5 minutes ..................................2
     More than 5 minutes........................................3
     Around 10 minutes...........................................4
     More than 10 minutes......................................5

58.  In your opinion what is the *main thing* that affects how long your
     doctor spends with you?

     The problem I go with........................................1
     The number of people waiting .......................2
     What mood the doctor is in .............................3

59.  When you see your doctor do you get the chance to say everything
     you want to say or not?

     Yes, always........................................................1
     Usually...............................................................2
     Sometimes..........................................................3
     Never ..................................................................4

60.  Do you feel that your doctor listens well to what you say or not?

     Listens well........................................................1
     Does not listen well..........................................2

61.  When you see your doctor do you feel you have enough time to
     discuss things fully or not?

     Yes.......................................................................1
     No ........................................................................2

62.  Do you feel able to ask your doctor questions or not?

     Can ask questions .............................................1
     Feel unable to ask questions ...........................2

63.  Does your doctor always examine you when you think it is
     necessary?

     Always ................................................................1
     Usually...............................................................2
     Sometimes..........................................................3
     Never ..................................................................4

64.  On the whole do you think your doctor gives you as much time and
     attention as you need?

     Yes.......................................................................1
     No ........................................................................2

65.  Have you ever put off seeing your doctor because you thought the
     doctor would not spend enough time with you?

     Yes.......................................................................1
     No ........................................................................2

The precise stages through which each module or batch of modules was put varied from topic to topic. For example, the module about patient–doctor communication (Seeing the doctor) was developed from a topic guide, the semi-structured version was tested by calling back on a quota sample of people completing it, and a pilot test was made with a structured version on a postal sample. For other topics, such as for home visits, the first stage was omitted.

**Performance of the modular questionnaires**

Results from the pilot and full-scale surveys using the modules illustrate some of the performance qualities of the questions and thus the potential usefulness of the information produced.

The achieved samples in each area were similar in terms of age and sex distributions. Answers differed according to age and sex but, since compared samples contain similar age/sex distributions, this means that one possible source of spurious variation in results from the surveys of different populations can be discounted. Responses to the surveys from different age groups (men and women) were remarkably consistent between the various areas.

*Reliability of questions*

Some idea of the reliability or repeatability of questions can be gained by use of the test–retest method. Here a variation of this method was used to assess the repeatability of questions.

Many of the questions that were tried in the larger scale pilots of modules 1 to 4 in the four FHSAs were retained for use in the full-scale surveys later carried out. Here results from 45 questions from these modules, which were either identical or very similar to each other in the questionnaire, are taken as illustrative. The results compared here are those from the pilot and full surveys in Salford FHSA.

Although sampling methods were similar (a random sample of those aged 16+ from the FHSA list), some discrepancy in results could be expected from differences in sample sizes between the pilots and full surveys. The Salford pilot size ranged from 88 to 138 responses according to question, the full-scale survey from 697 to 1,085 responses. Also, because the pilot sample was drawn from just one part of Salford it only included users of some, not all, Salford practices. Therefore questions that asked for descriptions of practice arrangements or reports of practice organisation were expected to show some differences.

The aim was to compare estimates obtained of the proportions giving specific responses using 95% confidence limits. If results from the two surveys fell within a similar error range they are referred to here as being in agreement. Results of this comparison were reassuring. Overall, results for 39 of the 45 questions compared were in agreement.

Questions were then divided into four broad categories. The first category contained 14 questions which asked people to report on their experiences of service delivery without an evaluation: for example, 'Does the receptionist ever ask you why you want to see the doctor?'. Of the 14 compared, 8 were in agreement, the rest producing estimates that were different at the 95% confidence level. The second category were questions that asked people for their evaluation of the service received: for example, 'Do you mind receptionists asking why you want to see the doctor?'. Twelve questions were in this category and all produced estimates that were not significantly different (at the 95% confidence level). The third category contained 10 questions asking users about their own behaviour or preferences: for example, 'Do you prefer to see your own doctor each time you go?'. All 10 produced estimates that were in agreement. The fourth category asked about people's characteristics or circumstances, for example their health status or housing tenure. Again all 9 sets of comparisons were in agreement.

Thus all those questions that produced results that were different ($p < 0.05$) were those particularly sensitive to differences in practice arrangements. Comparison of results for the sub-sample for the part of Salford surveyed in the pilot showed a high level of agreement.

We have therefore been able to show that the same question used at different times on two random samples from the same populations produced similar responses.

*Internal consistency*

Internal consistency is defined as the extent to which responses to sets of questions follow a predictable pattern. As an example, results for users' experience and opinions of appointment systems are compared here.

Three questions were compared: the first asked users to report how long they waited for their most recent appointment, the second whether this appointment was within the time they wanted, and the third whether or not they thought they should be able to get appointments more quickly. It was predicted that, where waits were shorter, more people would say they were within the time

**Table 3.** Comparison of responses about appointment systems.

|  | FHSA 'B' | FHSA 'A' | FHSA 'C' |
|---|---|---|---|
| Most recent appointment was for same or next day | 80% | 64% | 61% |
| This was within the time wanted | 86% | 78% | 75% |
| Appointments should be provided more quickly | 30% | 37% | 39% |

they wanted and fewer would say that appointments should be provided more quickly. Results for the three areas were compared and bore out these predictions (Table 3).

*Sensitivity of evaluative questions*

In addition to questions asking people to report experiences of service delivery, there were also questions that asked them to evaluate the acceptability of this performance. Here we have selected, as an illustrative example, two sets of results, one relating to appointment booking and the other to consultation times. The results here are for sub-samples of women aged 18–39 in each survey. In the Salford, Oldham and Tameside surveys, the same questions were asked about how long people had waited for their most recent appointment and a follow-up, and about whether this was within the time they wanted or not (Table 4). As already seen, there is a range in time waited, from those getting a 'same day' appointment to those having to wait longer than 3 days. Our concern was whether responses to the question about acceptability (within time wanted) reflected differences in the times waited.

We found an association between acceptability and delay in getting appointments ($p < 0.05$). Thus 93% of those in FHSA 'B'

**Table 4.** Percentage saying most recent appointment with preferred doctor was within time wanted; women 18–39.

|  | Same or next day | Day after next | Later |
|---|---|---|---|
| FHSA 'B' ($n = 200$) | 93% | 71% | 44% |
| FHSA 'A' ($n = 175$) | 86% | 74% | 47% |
| FHSA 'C' ($n = 273$) | 88% | 53% | 28% |

Tau-c ($p < 0.05$): 'B' 0.35; 'A' 0.32; 'C' 0.57

getting same/next day appointments said this was within the time they wanted, but only 44% of those waiting 3 days or more said this.

The nature of this relationship between time waited and acceptability was similar in three different surveys (measured using Kendall's tau, which gives a guide as to the strength of a relationship and not solely as to whether one existed or not).

*Duration of consultation and time to discuss problem*

People in the Salford and Oldham surveys were asked identical questions about how long their usual consultation lasted. This was followed by a question asking whether people had enough time to discuss things fully with their doctor. It was hoped that differences in response to this would reflect differences in duration of consultation. This did appear to be so: only about a third (in both areas) of those with consultations of less than 5 minutes said there was enough time whereas, amongst those who said their consultation lasted between 5 and 10 minutes, over 80% said that they had enough time.

## Illustrative results from the general practitioner surveys

The development work on the modules and their use in full-scale surveys mean that results are available for a wide range of aspects of general practitioner services. There are results for every item listed under the modules, and for some items there are results from the four FHSAs based on large samples (all more than 1,200 people, with response rates of 65–75%). This information has several uses:

- It shows the range of results for different aspects in different areas.
- It provides points of comparison for other surveys using the same questions.
- It shows what can be achieved in service delivery (in the 'best' cases).
- It shows those who are planning surveys what kind of response they might expect from particular modules or questions.

*Differences between FHSA areas*

Similar questions were used in full-scale surveys in Salford, Oldham and Tameside. Important differences between FHSAs emerged: for example, in FHSA 'A' only just over 1 in 10 people said that their general practitioner's surgery was sometimes closed during the day, whereas in FHSA 'C' over 1 in 3 said it closed during the day. In FHSA 'B' just over 1 in 10 had to wait 2 days or longer for an appointment with any doctor at the surgery, whereas nearly double that proportion had to wait this long in FHSA 'A'.

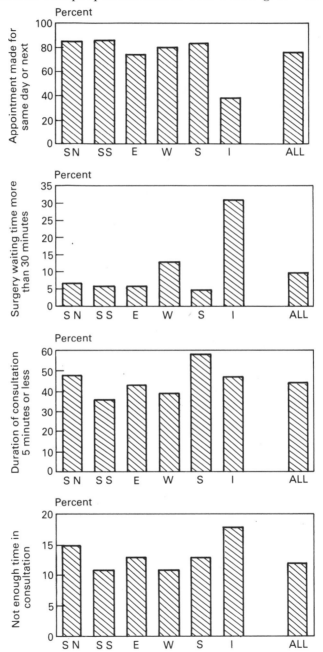

**Fig. 1.** *Variations in certain service aspects between different geographical areas of FHSA 'B'.*

## Differences within FHSA areas

One aspect that interested FHSAs was the variation in services within their districts. Responses for practices in different parts of the FHSA areas were grouped and compared. There were quite striking differences for some service aspects. For example, in FHSA 'B', practices in one part were much worse at providing early appointments and keeping people waiting when they came for their appointments. There were also differences in respect of consultation times (Fig. 1).

In FHSA 'C' nearly 4 out of 10 using practices in one part of the area said they waited more than 3 days for an appointment with their general practitioner; this compared with less than 1 in 10 kept waiting so long in two other parts of the area.

The availability of women doctors is an issue that concerns many. In FHSA 'C' the survey showed that no patients in one part and very few in another part of the area had a woman general practitioner, while in another part of the area more than a quarter had women general practitioners.

## Differences between sub-groups in the population

People in different circumstances have different needs and expectations from health services. It is important not to focus only on the global results of surveys. It has been shown often that age affects not only needs but also the evaluation of services. Our surveys showed similar differences. For example, younger respondents (16–39 years old) were more likely to report that they sometimes put off going to the general practitioner because they found surgery times inconvenient. Another example arises from a follow-up question to those respondents who said that receptionists asked them why they wanted appointments. About 60% of those aged 16–39 years said they disliked being asked their reasons, compared with just over 30% of the over-60s. Thus the large survey results can be broken down to highlight the particular problems faced by people with different needs.

## Purpose and uses of FHSA patient surveys

FHSAs have been encouraged to use consumer surveys to evaluate the services provided for them by their contracted professionals, but without much guidance as to the purposes for which they would be useful. Consumer satisfaction surveys are a relatively blunt instrument for informing policy making and implementation; they require careful advance planning for effective use.

The modules described in this report, and the questions within them, which have been developed and tested in field trials, provide FHSAs with tools for a variety of jobs that they need to do. They could be used for a baseline audit, which in turn could indicate the need for further audit or enquiry where less acceptable patterns of care were indicated. They may also be used for evaluation of policy changes, to identify perceived unmet needs in sub-groups of the population, or to identify perceived successes that could indicate good practice and provide the basis for enabling its widespread adoption.

Not only FHSAs need this sort of information; so do the contractors' professional organisations such as local medical committees. However, few of them have the resources to carry out population surveys of this sort. Thus, while they could be expected to be resistant to surveys for some of the above purposes, in other situations they might be expected to welcome the opportunity to cooperate in the design and analysis of such work.

While some have criticised these efforts as being no more than public relations exercises, FHSAs have legitimate concerns with responsibilities for planning services and monitoring the success of those plans. The surveys must address the real concerns of users and those who commission the survey, and the results must be trustworthy as a basis for action. Such surveys must therefore adhere to certain standards of formal research, and care must be taken to select appropriate modules, achieve representative and unbiased samples with high response rates, and use proper analytical techniques to elucidate the meaning of the results obtained.

Further details of the surveys and response rates and copies of the questionnaires can be obtained from the authors: Ralph Leavey and Alison Wilson, School of Health, St Martin's College, Lancaster LA1 3JD. An interim report is also available.[11]

## References

1. Cartwright A. *Patients and their doctors: a study of general practice.* London: Routledge and Kegan Paul, 1967.
2. Cartwright A, Anderson R. *General practice revisited: a second study of patients and their doctors.* London: Tavistock, 1981.
3. Ritchie J, Jacoby A, Bone M. *Access to primary health care.* London: HMSO, 1981.
4. Jacoby A. *User surveys of general practice: some findings from a postal survey of users' views and experiences of general practice.* London: Institute for Social Studies in Medical Care, 1989.

5. Consumers Association. *GP satisfaction survey report.* London: Consumers Association/Mass Observation, 1989.
6. Arber S, Sawyer L. *Changes in the structure of general practice: the patients' viewpoint.* Guildford: Department of Sociology, University of Surrey, 1979.
7. Leavey R. *Inequalities in urban primary care: use and acceptability of GP services.* Manchester: Centre for Primary Care Research, University of Manchester, 1983.
8. Leavey R. *Access to GPs: a fair share for all?* Manchester: Centre for Primary Care Research, University of Manchester, 1985.
9. Allen D, Leavey R, Marks B. Survey of patients' satisfaction with access to general practitioners. *Journal of the Royal College of General Practitioners* 1988; **38**: 163–5.
10. Prescott-Clarke P, Brooks T, Machray C. *Focus on health care. Surveying the public in four health districts.* Vol. 1: *The findings.* London: Social and Community Planning Research, Royal Institute of Public Administration, 1988.
11. Leavey R, Wilson AJ. Consumer surveys for family practitioner committees. *Department of Health Yearbook on Research and Development.* London: HMSO, 1990.

# 5 | Use of psychometrics to develop a measure of patient satisfaction for general practice

**Richard Baker**
*Eli Lilly National Medical Audit Centre, Department of General Practice, University of Leicester*

In common with other sectors of the health service, general practice has witnessed an explosion of interest in patient satisfaction. Whilst this is encouraging for those who wish to see a more equal relationship between doctors and patients, the rush to ask patients what they think has largely obscured the many questions about how patient opinion should be surveyed. Enthusiasm is not sufficient. There is already some suspicion about the value of surveys, and there must be a risk that the unthinking use of dubious survey methods will lead to the collection of questionable data. Over the past 3 years a programme to develop a measure for use by general practitioners has been undertaken in the general practice unit at the University of Bristol. The initial testing is complete and it is now being put to wider use in the South Western Regional Health Authority. In this chapter the development of the measure will be described.

## What is patient satisfaction?

Measurements are meaningless unless there is some concept of the object to be measured. In the case of patient satisfaction it is not entirely clear what is being measured. There is no widely accepted theory of what it is or what it means, so the development programme was based on a simple concept of satisfaction that could be employed until a more definitive theory has been widely agreed. One model for patient satisfaction with general practice has been devised by a working group of Liverpool Medical Audit Advisory Group.[1] They have suggested a three-level scheme: the first level is related to making contact with the service; the second is the way in which the doctor helps the patient with his or her illness; and the third is a reflection on the service and its effects on health status.

The social and psychological issues that underlie satisfaction are complex, and other models have been proposed that take these into account.[2-4] There is a common theme to these proposals. Satisfaction is an attitude that follows a process of judgement or cogitation upon experiences of the service. Previously held opinions and expectations may influence the judgement. When a patient is asked whether or not he or she is satisfied, the patient will pause for a moment and reflect on a potentially enormous list of events. These will include the difficulties experienced in getting an appointment, the inconvenience of taking time off work, the choice of doctor, the care given by the doctor, and the effectiveness of the treatment. All these issues will be viewed in the light of previous experiences of health care and expectations that have occurred. Personal characteristics such as attitudes to authority, beliefs about health and medicine, personality, age and sex may also play a role in modulating the formation of opinions. All these factors will be rapidly and largely unconsciously considered by the patient who will usually end up by summarising the answer with a 'yes, I am satisfied'. Satisfaction is first of all a summary. It is a brief description of so wide a range of experience and belief that it can hardly ever be other than simple acquiescence. How can such an amount of feeling be rolled up into a simple accurate statement? It is not surprising that satisfaction surveys so often report that 90% or more of patients say they are satisfied, because the language of satisfaction is too restricted to convey the many nuances of attitude. The real answer that patients give, if allowed, to the question 'Are you satisfied?' is more likely to be 'Yes, but I had to wait ages for an appointment' or 'Yes, but the doctor didn't tell me much about my illness'. If surveys of satisfaction are to be useful they must uncover the 'but' part of answers. The main feature of the model of satisfaction that I adopted in the development of measuring instruments was that satisfaction was a summary, and the aim was to encourage patients to express their 'buts'.

## Types of instrument

There are three main methods that can be used to measure patient opinion. Because these can overlap, and because they are sometimes used indiscriminately, it can appear that there are many methods. However, it is usually possible to place a survey into one of three categories.

The first is the *ad hoc* survey. General practitioners in a practice may wish to ask patients what they think about a particular aspect of their service. This survey is a tool to aid practice management. A short list of questions is selected and submitted to a sample of patients. Whilst this type of survey has many technical deficiencies, it does serve a purpose, that of giving some guidance to a practice facing a specific problem. The method is easy, perhaps too easy, and many examples have been reported, but it is inappropriate to generalise from the findings.

There are reputable methods for investigating opinions that can be used when the topic of interest is of more general importance. These methods allow conclusions to be drawn based on robust evidence. They can be used for management and research. The methods are either qualitative or quantitative. In general practice in this country the qualitative survey has a long and distinguished record. Surveys of this kind can be used to identify issues that are important to patients when they make their judgements about care. A number of techniques can be used, such as extended interviews which can be recorded on to tape for future analysis by coding. The degree of structuring of the interview can vary. A questionnaire can be used with a large proportion of closed questions, but also with the facility to record the respondent's clarifications and explanations, or an almost unstructured interview can be used that follows the respondent's individual concerns using open questions. This kind of survey demands a great deal of skill in both execution and analysis. Whilst essential information can be uncovered and depicted in pinpoint clarity using respondents' own words, the investment of time, skill and money can be considerable.

Whilst qualitative surveys can identify the constituents of patient satisfaction, quantitative surveys can be used to measure them. The development of quantitative survey methods is no less skilled than that for qualitative surveys, but once developed they can often be used with only limited expertise. The methods have been borrowed from the science of psychometrics, a branch of psychology concerned with the measurement of traits such as personality or intelligence. It is a method for measuring qualities for which there is no physical scale. Quantitative surveys are more amenable than qualitative surveys to statistical tests of reliability and validity. Their properties can be precisely delineated in order to show when their use is or is not appropriate and how much reliance should be placed on the findings. In this respect they can be compared with laboratory investigations when a particular result has to be interpreted in the light of the qualities of the test itself. In the field of health care there is an increasing appreciation of the potential of psychometrics as one approach to measuring the outcome of care, and a substantial number of scales have been devised for the measurement of health status. Examples of psychometrics applied to the measurement of patient satisfaction are less common. One of the earliest such instruments was developed by Ware and colleagues in North America in the 1970s.[5-7]. Their patient satisfaction questionnaire was designed to be a self-administered measure that could be used in a general population for the evaluation of services. The final version of the questionnaire comprised 68 questions divided into a number of sub-scales including access to care, financial aspects, technical quality and overall satisfaction. The questionnaire was thoroughly tested and the results demonstrated that it is possible to develop measures of satisfaction that are reliable, valid and produce easily understood scores. It has since been used extensively and is the model I have followed in the development of the questionnaires reported here.

## Aims for the questionnaires

When the development of the questionnaires in this project began there was a clear need for measures of the outcome of care including patient satisfaction.[8] The ideal measure would be easy for general practitioners to use in their own practices and would enable comparison to be made between doctors and practices. If general practitioners can see how they compare with their peers, they will have a clear picture of what parts of their service could be improved. Whilst no two practices are exactly the same, the measure should be applicable in the vast majority. As many aspects of care as possible should be included, but at the same time the measure should be flexible in use and not impose an unreasonable burden on respondents. The measure should be focused on general practice rather than on primary care services. The addition of questions about community or hospital services would make it unacceptably long, and only a small proportion of patients would have enough experience of the health service to answer every question. The measure should have high levels of reliability and validity in order to ensure that users have confidence in the findings. General practitioners are unlikely to be encouraged to make changes in their practices on the evidence of questionable data. These specifications pointed to psychometrics as the preferred method.

General practice cares for people at all stages of the human life cycle, and with all clinical and psychosocial conditions. The range of activities that a practice can undertake is consequently considerable. In order to meet the specifications, some aspects of care were not included. For example, patient views on home visits were omitted. Questions about home visits administered to a patient who has not recently requested one will irritate the respondent and will produce answers of dubious value. Likewise questions about referral to secondary care or attendance at special practice sessions such as antenatal or health promotional clinics would extend the length of the proposed questionnaire and not be applicable to many patients and some practices. It was therefore decided to concentrate on the two ineluctable features of practice—the consultation and the facilities that allow the consultation to take place. To aid flexibility of use and limit the length of questionnaire, two questionnaires were planned, one concerned with the consultation (the consultation satisfaction questionnaire, CSQ) and the other concerned with opinions on the practice as a whole (the surgery satisfaction questionnaire, SSQ).* Depending on the experience gained from these questionnaires, further versions may be developed for use in specific situations such as special clinics or referral to outpatient departments.

## Identifying the issues

The first step in the development of the questionnaire was to identify those areas of care that are of concern to patients. The questionnaires should contain questions about each of these topics in order to contribute to content validity. There is an extensive literature in the field of patient opinion about general practice. Many qualitative studies have been undertaken by medical sociologists and others, including journalists, and these give important guidance to the issues that patients use to reach their judgements on satisfaction. These studies confirm that satisfaction is not a simple unitary concept but is a composite or summary of a series of views on different aspects of care. The review of the literature on general practice was supplemented by examination of the contents of other satisfaction questionnaires. A third source of patient opinion was personal experience of the comments patients themselves make about services. For example, patients will sometimes tell the general practitioner about the difficulties of making an appointment or that the telephone is always engaged on Monday mornings. Receptionists, nurses and other team members are also the recipients of comments on what the patient thinks of the doctor. A patient participation group is active in the practice in which most of the development work was undertaken. From all these sources, a library of possible questions was devised. The original list contained 135 questions about the surgery in general and 126 about the consultation.

---

* The general practitioner's surgery is the equivalent of the physician's office in the USA.

The style chosen was that of a statement followed by five possible answers ranging from strong agreement to strong disagreement. Questions in this format allow for a range of opinion to be expressed and can be used to calculate a score. This is the familiar five-point Likert scale.[9] A five-point scale was selected because this is simple and familiar to many people and so should be relatively straightforward for most respondents. As some respondents will have no opinions either way on some topics, the mid-point in the scale was classified as 'neutral'. An additional source of potential questions was provided by the inclusion of two open questions on the first pilot test of each questionnaire, to catch any topics of concern to patients that had not been covered. These open questions asked if there was anything the patient particularly liked or disliked about the surgery or the doctor. Extra comments expressed by patients did not in the event turn up any useful new questions. There were some comments about the surgery car park entrance, a problem only encountered in the main test surgery and therefore inappropriate in the evaluation of other surgeries, and the comment that the doctor was a good listener. When a question about the doctor listening was included in later field tests, the response was highly positively skewed, indicating that it discriminated badly between different levels of satisfaction. This does not mean that the underlying doctor behaviour of being a 'good listener' is not important, just that the direct question is not useful. In the final version of the consultation questionnaire, questions that reflected the *consequences* of being a good listener, such as those about knowing the patient well or the patient feeling able to tell the doctor very personal things, were better at obtaining a range of replies.

## Refinement of the questionnaire

Once possible questions had been identifed they were given to patients in a number of field trials; the experience of these directed improvements. The most simple evaluation was review of questions to check for ambiguity or other problems. Respondents will sometimes write comments on the questionnaire to say that a question is difficult to understand. Colleagues were shown the questionnaires and asked for their comments. Patients who show a socially desirable set of responses give answers that they feel are the most acceptable rather than what they feel; care must be taken to avoid this. Another procedure was to plot the distribution of replies to each question in order to identify questions that did not produce a range of response. Particularly skewed questions have not discriminated between different levels of satisfaction and are not acceptable measures (see Chapter 2). The distribution of responses to one question used in an early field trial is shown in Fig. 1. When the question was phrased in a different way the response lost its skewed distribution (Fig. 2). By no means all the

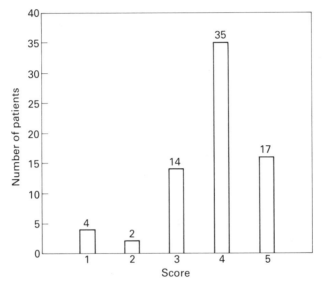

**Fig. 1.** *Responses in field trial 2 of the CSQ to the question: 'This doctor doesn't know how I feel'.*

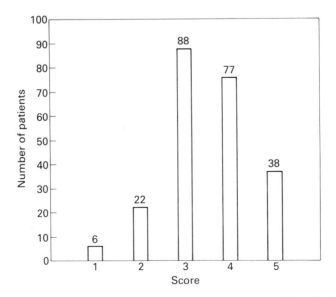

**Fig. 2.** *Responses in field trial 6 of the CSQ to the question: 'I felt this doctor really knew what I was thinking'.*

questions that have been retained in the final versions of the questionnaires have ideal normal distributions, although some progress was made in changing the phrasing of questions to encourage patients to express negative opinions. In attempting to overcome response bias, there is a danger that repeatedly modifying questions leads to such bland phraseology that the questions become meaningless; in other words, they could lose face validity. The final questions were a balance between these competing requirements.

From the third field trial onwards, an additional statistical procedure was used to aid test development. Principal components analysis (PCA)[10] is a method that calculates how each question is answered relative to the others and then throws these correlations into multidimensional space. The questions can be imagined as a group of planets in space. The procedure then draws into this space the axes that best fit the distribution of the questions or planets. These axes are the components. There are a number of mathematical ways by which the best fit can be calculated. In the development of the questionnaires a method called Varimax rotation was used. One purpose of PCA is to reveal those questions that do not lie within reasonable distance of an axis. If a question is floating unconnected with a particular theme, it is either asking patients about very little, perhaps because the question is poorly worded, ambiguous or highly skewed in response, or alternatively it is about an important topic but there are no other questions on the subject. Review of the questions shows which explanation is correct. For example, the fourth field test of the consultation questionnaire showed only two components. Questions about interpersonal aspects of the consultation had been omitted, a deficiency that was remedied in the fifth field trial.

Questions grouped together can be used to produce an amalgamated score for the theme or component. By using several questions to check on the patient's view of a broad topic such as quality of the premises, reliability is increased and greater weight can be placed on the findings. Use of multi-item scales in this way rather than single-item questions helps to make quantitative measures more robust.

The component structures of the sixth and final version of both questionnaires are available from the author. The correlation matrix of the fifth version of SSQ has been reported,[11] and the structure of the sixth version is the same except for the addition of nine new questions. The sixth version of each questionnaire is included in this chapter. Some questions are worded positively and some negatively. In order to calculate a score for each component of care, the direction of scores must be taken into account. The

**Table 1.** Question numbers for each component of satisfaction, showing whether they were worded positively (score 1 for strongly disagree, 5 for strongly agree) or negatively (score 5 for strongly disagree, 1 for strongly agree). Also shown are the calculations to convert the component total scores into standardised scores with a maximum of 100 for each component. The questionnaires and the numbering of the questions are shown on pages 66–69.

| Component | Questions worded positively | Questions worded negatively | Conversion to 100 scale ($x$ = sum of question scores) |
|---|---|---|---|
| **SSQ** | | | |
| General satisfaction | 1,24 | 12 | $x \times 100/15$ |
| Accessibility | 14 | 4, 10, 21 | $x \times 100/20$ |
| Availability | 18 | 6, 13, 17, 22 | $x \times 100/25$ |
| Continuity | 3, 26 | 9, 15, 20 | $x \times 100/25$ |
| Medical care | 5, 8, 11 | 23 | $x \times 100/25$ |
| Premises | 7 | 2, 16, 19, 25 | $x \times 100/25$ |
| **CSQ** | | | |
| General satisfaction | 1 | 7, 17 | $x \times 100/15$ |
| Professional care | 2, 3, 6, 9, 10, 12, 13 | | $x \times 100/35$ |
| Depth of relationship | 4, 14,15 | 8, 18 | $x \times 100/25$ |
| Perceived length of consultation | | 5, 11, 16 | $x \times 100/15$ |

direction of each question is shown in Table 1. A score of 1 indicates dissatisfaction, and 5 satisfaction. To make understanding even easier, the scores for each component are converted arithmetically on to a scale with a maximum score of 100 for each component. Details are shown in Table 1.

## Reliability

Tests of reliability determine whether the questionnaires are measuring satisfaction in a reproducible and consistent fashion. The definition of reliability is the ratio of true variance between subjects to the true variance plus or minus the variance due to error.[12] This may be calculated in a number of ways, including analysis of variance. Two methods have been used to assess the reliabilities of SSQ and CSQ.

**SSQ**                                                                            **CONFIDENTIAL**

**UNIVERSITY OF BRISTOL**
**GENERAL PRACTICE UNIT**
**DEPARTMENT OF EPIDEMIOLOGY & PUBLIC HEALTH MEDICINE**

**SURGERY SATISFACTION QUESTIONNAIRE**

The questions on this form ask you what you think of your surgery and the care you receive. Please answer every question on each page of the form. Your answers will be kept entirely confidential so do not write your name on the form. Please be sure to place this form in the box provided before you leave today.

The questions are set out in the same way. **For each one draw a circle round the answer that is closest to what you think.** "Neutral" means you have no feelings either way.

For example:
"This surgery is too big."                Strongly Agree/Agree/Neutral/Disagree/Strongly Disagree

---

1.  I am totally satisfied
    with everything about this          Strongly Agree/Agree/Neutral/Disagree/Strongly Disagree
    general practice

2.  I do not much like my
    surgery's waiting room              Strongly Agree/Agree/Neutral/Disagree/Strongly Disagree

3.  I see the same doctor
    almost every time I go              Strongly Agree/Agree/Neutral/Disagree/Strongly Disagree
    to the surgery

4.  It can take me a long time
    to get to my doctor's surgery       Strongly Agree/Agree/Neutral/Disagree/Strongly Disagree

5.  The doctors at this surgery
    are always careful not to           Strongly Agree/Agree/Neutral/Disagree/Strongly Disagree
    make any mistakes

6.  It can be difficult to get
    through to the surgery              Strongly Agree/Agree/Neutral/Disagree/Strongly Disagree
    on the telephone

7.  My doctor's surgery is modern
    and up to date                      Strongly Agree/Agree/Neutral/Disagree/Strongly Disagree

8.  I am always satisfied with the
    medical care I receive              Strongly Agree/Agree/Neutral/Disagree/Strongly Disagree
    at this surgery

9.  It can be difficult to see the
    same doctor each time you           Strongly Agree/Agree/Neutral/Disagree/Strongly Disagree
    go to the surgery

10. I find this surgery very
    difficult to get to                 Strongly Agree/Agree/Neutral/Disagree/Strongly Disagree

11. The doctors at this surgery
    never make mistakes                 Strongly Agree/Agree/Neutral/Disagree/Strongly Disagree

12. I am not completely satisfied
    with one or two things about        Strongly Agree/Agree/Neutral/Disagree/Strongly Disagree
    this general practice

**Please turn over**

13. It can be hard to get an
    appointment for medical        Strongly Agree/Agree/Neutral/Disagree/Strongly Disagree
    care right away

14. My doctor's surgery is
    very easy to get to            Strongly Agree/Agree/Neutral/Disagree/Strongly Disagree

15. I do not always see the same
    doctor when I go to the surgery Strongly Agree/Agree/Neutral/Disagree/Strongly Disagree

16. This surgery building could
    do with some improvements      Strongly Agree/Agree/Neutral/Disagree/Strongly Disagree

17. It can sometimes be difficult
    to get an appointment at
    this surgery                   Strongly Agree/Agree/Neutral/Disagree/Strongly Disagree

18. They always answer the telephone
    straightaway at this surgery   Strongly Agree/Agree/Neutral/Disagree/Strongly Disagree

19. I think this surgery building
    could be a little better       Strongly Agree/Agree/Neutral/Disagree/Strongly Disagree

20. I wish it was easier to see
    my own doctor every time       Strongly Agree/Agree/Neutral/Disagree/Strongly Disagree
    I go to the surgery

21. Travelling to the surgery
    can be a problem to me         Strongly Agree/Agree/Neutral/Disagree/Strongly Disagree

22. Getting an appointment when
    you want one can sometimes     Strongly Agree/Agree/Neutral/Disagree/Strongly Disagree
    be a little difficult

23. I think the medical care at
    this surgery could sometimes   Strongly Agree/Agree/Neutral/Disagree/Strongly Disagree
    be better

24. I am satisfied with most things
    about this general practice    Strongly Agree/Agree/Neutral/Disagree/Strongly Disagree

25. This surgery building should
    be improved to make it more    Strongly Agree/Agree/Neutral/Disagree/Strongly Disagree
    pleasant inside

26. There are never any problems in
    seeing the same doctor each time Strongly Agree/Agree/Neutral/Disagree/Strongly Disagree
    you go to the surgery


How old are you?                                    _____    years

Are you male          _____        or female    _____    (Tick which applies)


THANK YOU FOR COMPLETING THIS QUESTIONNAIRE

CSQ                                                                    **CONFIDENTIAL**

**GENERAL PRACTICE UNIT**
**UNIVERSITY OF BRISTOL**
**DEPARTMENT OF EPIDEMIOLOGY & PUBLIC HEALTH MEDICINE**

**CONSULTATION SATISFACTION QUESTIONNAIRE**

This form contains a list of questions. They ask you what you think of your last visit to the doctor. Please answer all the questions. Your answers will be kept entirely confidential and will not be shown to the doctor so feel free to say what you wish. Please do not write your name on the form and be sure to place this form in the box provided before you leave today.

For each question circle the answer that is closest to what you think. "Neutral" means you have no feelings either way.

For example:

"This doctor was bored"                    Strongly Agree/Agree/(Neutral)/Disagree/Strongly Disagree

---

1.    I am totally satisfied
      with my visit to this doctor        Strongly Agree/Agree/Neutral/Disagree/Strongly Disagree

2.    This doctor was very careful
      to check everything when             Strongly Agree/Agree/Neutral/Disagree/Strongly Disagree
      examining me

3.    I will follow this doctor's
      advice because I think               Strongly Agree/Agree/Neutral/Disagree/Strongly Disagree
      he/she is absolutely right

4.    I felt able to tell this doctor
      about very personal things           Strongly Agree/Agree/Neutral/Disagree/Strongly Disagree

5.    The time I was able to spend
      with the doctor was a bit            Strongly Agree/Agree/Neutral/Disagree/Strongly Disagree
      too short

6.    This doctor told me
      everything about my                  Strongly Agree/Agree/Neutral/Disagree/Strongly Disagree
      treatment

7.    Some things about my
      consultation with the doctor         Strongly Agree/Agree/Neutral/Disagree/Strongly Disagree
      could have been better

8.    There are some things this
      doctor does not know                 Strongly Agree/Agree/Neutral/Disagree/Strongly Disagree
      about me

**Please turn over**

9.    This doctor examined me very
      thoroughly                          Strongly Agree/Agree/Neutral/Disagree/Strongly Disagree

10.   I thought this doctor took
      notice of me as a person            Strongly Agree/Agree/Neutral/Disagree/Strongly Disagree

11.   The time I was allowed to
      spend with the doctor was           Strongly Agree/Agree/Neutral/Disagree/Strongly Disagree
      not long enough to deal with
      everything I wanted

12.   I understand my illness much
      better after seeing this doctor     Strongly Agree/Agree/Neutral/Disagree/Strongly Disagree

13.   This doctor was interested
      in me as a person not               Strongly Agree/Agree/Neutral/Disagree/Strongly Disagree
      just my illness

14.   This doctor knows all
      about me                            Strongly Agree/Agree/Neutral/Disagree/Strongly Disagree

15.   I felt this doctor really knew
      what I was thinking                 Strongly Agree/Agree/Neutral/Disagree/Strongly Disagree

16.   I wish it had been possible to
      spend a little longer with          Strongly Agree/Agree/Neutral/Disagree/Strongly Disagree
      the doctor

17.   I am not completely satisfied
      with my visit to the doctor         Strongly Agree/Agree/Neutral/Disagree/Strongly Disagree

18.   I would find it difficult to tell
      this doctor about some              Strongly Agree/Agree/Neutral/Disagree/Strongly Disagree
      private things


      How old are you?                                  _____ years


      Are you male  _____      or female   _____ (Tick which applies)



                    THANK YOU FOR COMPLETING THIS QUESTIONNAIRE

**Table 2.** Coefficient alpha internal consistency reliability coefficients for SSQ ($n = 983$) and CSQ ($n = 645$). The patients were from two general practices who had all been registered with their practice for at least two years.

| Component of satisfaction | Coefficient alpha |
| --- | --- |
| **SSQ** | |
| General satisfaction | 0.87 |
| Accessibility | 0.91 |
| Availability | 0.83 |
| Continuity | 0.89 |
| Medical care | 0.87 |
| Premises | 0.92 |
| **CSQ** | |
| General satisfaction | 0.91 |
| Professional care | 0.95 |
| Depth of relationship | 0.88 |
| Perceived length of consultation | 0.90 |

A test–retest study of reliability has been undertaken. Patients were mailed SSQ and CSQ twice 2 weeks apart; 131 completed and returned the questionnaires. The reliability was calculated using both analysis of variance and Pearson product moment coefficients; the findings are reported elsewhere.[13] The levels of reliability were all high. Similar levels of reliability have been obtained using a test of internal consistency, Cronbach's alpha.[14] This test requires only one administration of the questionnaires. The results are split in half and the halves compared, alpha being the mean of all possible such split half correlations. Alpha for CSQ and for the earlier version of SSQ have been reported.[11,15] Table 2 shows alpha for the latest versions of the questionnaires, calculated from a total of 983 responders for SSQ and 645 for CSQ who were mailed the questionnaires. This study was undertaken as part of a study of construct validity. In summary, both test–retest and internal consistency studies of reliability have shown that SSQ and CSQ have excellent levels of reliability.

## Validity

Evidence about the validity of the questionnaires comes from a variety of sources. Content validity is supported by the finding that the questionnaires do include questions about the topics most often identified as important to patients when they make judgements of care. No significant additional factors have been reported. Questions about receptionists were included on earlier versions of SSQ but these failed to discriminate. The impression was that patients do not judge receptionists separately. If the appointment system is effective and the availability of doctors adequate, patients are happy with the receptionists. However, if availability is not adequate the receptionists are viewed less favourably. A similar situation arose in patients' assessments of communication within the consultation. Here direct judgements about communication, eg the doctor being considered a 'good listener', proved unhelpful. Questions were more likely to obtain a range of response when the consequences of communication were considered, for example the patient's understanding of the illness and the doctor's apparent ability to know what the patient is thinking. Quality assurance traditionally divides care into technical and interpersonal aspects, and this is reflected in the components 'professional care' and 'depth of relationship'. Patients appear to expect that the ability to communicate information about the illness and treat the patient with respect are aspects of professional behaviour. They presume that doctors will examine them, explain about the illness and its treatment, and address them in a civilised manner. General practice has long been interested in the relationship between the doctor and the patient. Dating from the 1950s and the work of Michael Balint, the doctor has been considered as an important therapeutic instrument regardless of medication or other treatments. Patients do appear to value the depth of relationship they have with their doctors. Initially I felt some reluctance to name this component of satisfaction as 'depth of relationship' since this has many resonances within general practice. There are often said to be some things that cannot be measured. However, on discussing this component with colleagues, the consensus was that it was indeed about the relationship. Besides measuring this sensitive aspect of practice, the relationship of this component to previous work and the philosophy of general practice gives strong support to the contention that the questionnaires do have content validity.

Further evidence is provided by the correlations of each component of satisfaction with general satisfaction. The components of CSQ and SSQ should be related to general satisfaction. If they are not so related they cannot be claimed to be part of the overall construct or theory of satisfaction. The relationship should not be too strong; if levels of correlation are high the components may be measuring virtually the same thing as general satisfaction, and so

**Table 3.** Scores for SSQ and CSQ at different levels of continuity of care and for patients who changed surgeries without changing their home addresses. The method of calculating continuity of care is explained in the text.

| Component of satisfaction | Levels of continuity | | | | Patients changing doctors |
|---|---|---|---|---|---|
| | 100% | 75% | 50% | 25% | |
| **SSQ** | | | | | |
| Number of patients | 57 | 77 | 62 | 44 | 458 |
| General satisfaction | 81.5 | 79.6 | 67.5 | 67.3 | 52.9 |
| Accessibility | 79.4 | 80.1 | 76.7 | 77.5 | 62.4 |
| Availability | 66.4 | 65.5 | 53.5 | 58.4 | 53.9 |
| Continuity | 80.2 | 69.9 | 56.1 | 49.4 | 54.5 |
| Medical care | 80.1 | 77.7 | 66.1 | 65.3 | 54.3 |
| Premises | 82.9 | 79.4 | 76.3 | 73.6 | 59.2 |
| **CSQ** | | | | | |
| Number of patients | 43 | 47 | 38 | 20 | 264 |
| General satisfaction | 78.3 | 81.7 | 73.5 | 71.3 | 52.1 |
| Professional care | 79.9 | 80.3 | 73.4 | 70.3 | 56.2 |
| Depth of relationship | 72.3 | 74.8 | 62.3 | 60.4 | 53.8 |
| Perceived length of consultation | 71.3 | 76.4 | 72.3 | 68.0 | 54.6 |

not providing any additional information. Correlation scores between the components of satisfaction and the general satisfaction scale have been reported; all are in the range 0.2–0.6,[11,15] indicating that the components are related to general satisfaction but are not identical with it.

A test of criterion validity has been conducted using an earlier version of SSQ.[11] The scores from SSQ when given to 100 patients in each of eight surgeries were compared with the assessments of the surgeries made by an external assessor and by the doctors who worked at the surgeries. This was a test of whether the views of patients as revealed by the questionnaires were a valid judgement of quality. This was a demanding test as the questionnaires could be a valid measure of what the patients think of the surgeries, but patient opinions need not necessarily be valid judgements of quality. Nevertheless reassuring results were obtained, with validity coefficients of between 0.44 and 0.80 for the comparison of SSQ scores and the external assessor's judgement.

A study of construct validity has recently been completed[13] and this gives further evidence in support of the questionnaires' reliability. Patients attending two general practices were mailed SSQ and CSQ and the scores were compared with the scores of patients who changed surgeries without changing their home addresses. Only a small proportion of patients change surgeries without moving home, but there is evidence that those who do change are dissatisfied with the surgery they are leaving. It is a usual finding that patients who are dissatisfied are likely to switch providers, and this is part of the accepted construct of patient satisfaction. If CSQ and SSQ are valid they should classify these patients in different groups. The questionnaires performed exactly as the construct predicted. Some results from this study are shown in Table 3. The scores in the two groups are clearly different. Moreover, the questionnaires were sufficiently sensitive to demonstrate different scores for some components when the level of continuity experienced by patients varied. Continuity was calculated as the proportion of consultations out of twelve that were with the usual doctor. For most components of satisfaction, scores tended to decline as continuity declined.

**Transferability**

The transferability of a test is the degree to which it can be used in different types of population yet remain reliable and valid. Information about the transferability of CSQ and SSQ is so far limited, although experience is rapidly accumulating. The questionnaires have been used by patients in a range of practices, including several in the south west of England and some in the North of England. Large numbers of patients from low social classes have yet to use the questionnaires. There is also no experience of their use in ethnic minority populations. It may be more appropriate to develop different questionnaires altogether for these groups, as their members may judge health services in a different manner. For example, availability and accessibility may be less important than the religion or sex of the doctor.

**Range of scores**

The questionnaires do reveal a range of scores. This is confirmed by Table 3. This may reflect the care taken in questionnaire development to devise questions that did obtain a reasonable distribution of replies. The satisfaction scores for a large sample of doctors or surgeries have yet to be described. Whilst there is a wide difference between patients who change doctors without moving home and those who always return to see the same doctor, the difference between the highest and lowest scoring doctors and surgeries is unknown. Information about this will become available over the next year. A service has been made available to general practitioners in the South West Health Region to enable them to survey their patients' opinions using SSQ and CSQ. Approximately 100 practices will take part. Initial findings have shown that scores do differ in a logical way between practices. For example, practices in buildings that doctors themselves judge to be inadequate have lower satisfaction scores for premises. Future studies should attempt to depict the range of scores for practices in different parts of the country, in inner-city or suburban locations, and for different types of doctors. The characteristics of doctors that are related to patient satisfaction can be studied using CSQ. Women patients attending women doctors may report levels of satisfaction different from those of women attending men doctors. The effects of vocational training, membership of the Royal College of General Practitioners, and doctors' ages may all have some effect on patient satisfaction.

## Age and sex of respondents

We found that older patients report consistently higher levels of satisfaction, but sex proved to be unrelated to satisfaction.

## Conclusion

The original aim of this project was to develop questionnaires that general practitioners could use themselves. The tasks that remain to be completed before this is achieved are to detail the range of scores more completely and to produce a user's manual. The survey of 100 practices in the South West Health Region will supply sufficient experience to complete these tasks. The questionnaires will then be available for general practitioners to use in their own practices.

A series of studies have shown that the instruments have excellent reliability and validity in the conditions in which they have been used. Further information about transferability to other settings is required. They have a variety of potential uses, including audit of individual practices or by medical audit advisory groups. Family Health Service Authorities might also wish to evaluate satisfaction with general practitioner services throughout their localities. Findings from CSQ could be used to guide education in consultation skills, especially when combined with video recording of consultations. There are many questions about outcome and patient satisfaction that might be studied in research using the questionnaire. I hope that they will contribute to an increased understanding between doctors and their patients. This understanding is the basis for the therapeutic relationship.

## References

1. Liverpool Medical Audit Advisory Group. *How was it for you? Thinking about satisfaction with services.* Liverpool: Liverpool MAAG, Liverpool FHSA and Department of General Practice, University of Liverpool, 1991.
2. Linder-Pelz S. Toward a theory of patient satisfaction. *Social Science and Medicine* 1982; **16:** 577–82.
3. Locker D, Dunt D. Theoretical and methodological issues in sociological studies of consumer satisfaction with medical care. *Social Science and Medicine* 1978; **12:** 283–92.
4. Calnan M. Towards a conceptual framework of lay evaluation of health care. *Social Science and Medicine* 1988; **27:** 927–33.
5. Ware JE, Davies-Avery A, Stewart AL. The measurement and meaning of patient satisfaction. *Health and Medical Care Review* 1978;**1:** 2–15.
6. Ware JE, Snyder MK, Wright WR, Davies AR. Defining and measuring patient satisfaction with medical care. *Evaluation and Program Planning* 1983; **6:** 247–63.
7. Ware JE. How to survey patient satisfaction. *Drug Intelligence and Clinical Pharmacy* 1981; **15:** 892–9.
8. Baker R. *Practice assessment and quality of care.* Occasional Paper 39. London: Royal College of General Practitioners, 1988.
9. Likert R. A technique for the measurement of attitudes. *Archives of Psychology* (New York) 1932; **140:** 44–53.
10. Manley BFJ. *Multivariate statistical methods: a primer.* London: Chapman and Hall, 1986.
11. Baker R. The reliability and criterion validity of a measure of patients' satisfaction with their general practice. *Family Practice* 1991; **8:** 171–7.
12. Streiner DL, Norman GR. *Health measurement scales: a practical guide to their development and use.* Oxford: Oxford University Press, 1989.
13. Baker R, Whitfield M. Measuring patient satisfaction: a test of construct validity. *Quality in Health Care* 1992; **1:** 104–9.
14. McKennell A. Attitude measurement: use of coefficient alpha with cluster or factor analysis. In: Brynner J, Stribley KM, eds. *Social research: principles and procedures.* London: Longman, 1979.
15. Baker R. Development of a questionnaire to assess patients' satisfaction with consultations in general practice. *British Journal of General Practice* 1990; **40:** 487–90.

# 6 | Patient satisfaction in relation to clinical care: a neglected contribution

**Ray Fitzpatrick**
*Department of Public Health and Primary Care,*
*University of Oxford*
**Anthony Hopkins**
*Research Unit, Royal College of Physicians, London*

The main focus of patient satisfaction surveys in this country has been in areas such as the quality of hospital amenities and the accessibility of health care. There have been a small number of surveys in primary care which have extended their scope to include feedback from patients in such issues as the quality of medical care. In the hospital sector it is less common for surveys to stray beyond the so-called 'hotel' aspects of care. This can partly be explained in terms of the fact that enthusiasm for consumer surveys was generated by the Griffiths report on NHS management. Patient feedback is most naturally sought by managers with regard to those topics in which they feel most competent to intervene. Managers still sense that more core clinical aspects of health care are territories into which they may not stray—a view not discouraged by the medical profession.[1] As a result it is still largely true that managers conduct consumer satisfaction surveys and the medical profession conducts medical audit.[2]

Compared with their general practice colleagues, hospital-based doctors have seen less to gain from incorporating the patient's perspective into the process of audit or evaluation. There are exceptions to this observation,[3] and the value of the patient's viewpoint is to some extent recognised and applied in the form of the recently developed array of 'subjective health status' or 'quality of life' measures.[4] It is beyond the scope of this chapter to consider possible reasons for the different levels of interest in the assessment of patient satisfaction between primary and secondary health care. This chapter considers one particular study that set out to examine patient satisfaction in a hospital specialist clinic. In addition to reporting some results from the study, the chapter considers methodological advantages to assessing satisfaction in conjunction with detailed attention to the variety of concerns and expectations patients have about their health problem. We argue that patients' perceptions of health care are better understood, and ultimately make more important contributions to the evaluation of health care outcomes, if they are related to their views regarding their health problems.

## Referral to a neurologist for chronic headache

This chapter presents results from a study that the two editors carried out to examine the expectations and subsequent satisfaction with care of patients referred to neurologists with a primary presenting problem of headache.[5] It is unusual for a general practitioner to need specialist assistance in the management of headache. There may be some difficulty in distinguishing between such common problems as tension headache and migraine, or the general practitioner wishes the possibility of a more serious diagnosis such as a brain tumour to be considered. More recently a number of specialist clinics have been set up to provide more active advice and treatment for patients with migraine. Even if the neurologist is not involved in such a migraine clinic, he or she may receive a number of referrals in which specialist advice in the treatment of migraine is sought. Neurologists generally play a fairly limited role in the management of patients presenting with headache. They view their main task as providing a differential diagnosis (either to rule out structural lesions or to distinguish between, for example, migraine and tension headache) and, where appropriate, to advise about drug therapy. Occasional doubt had been expressed about the value of neurological referral for headache,[6] and a study was set up to examine the issue from the point of view of the patient.

## Recruitment and interviewing

A detailed account of methods of recruiting the sample and of the sample's social and medical characteristics is not relevant to this chapter and can be found elsewhere.[7] A sample of 95 patients was recruited, of whom 69% were women, with an average age of 37 and a range of social backgrounds. None of the patients eventually proved to have a serious lesion; most patients' symptoms were diagnosed as either 'tension headache' or 'migraine'. The sample's headaches closely resembled in severity those reported for other clinic studies.[8] As in other clinic surveys,[9] most patients (67%) reported that their headaches had been a problem for more than a year.

Non-schedule standardised interviews[10] were used and were tape-recorded. Patients were first recruited and then interviewed at the hospital clinic prior to their consultation with the neurologist. The focus of this interview was on the patient's perception of the problem and on expectations of clinic attendance. In a second and much longer interview, conducted in the patient's home 2–3 weeks after the hospital visit, a detailed account was obtained of the patient's history of coping with headaches and of perceptions and evaluations of the hospital visit.

The type of interview used is standardised in the sense that the interviewer wishes to obtain a standardised set of data from each respondent, but there is no fixed schedule of set questions used to obtain the data. The interviewer thus has a clear view of ultimate objectives to be achieved, but the interview may be quite interactive and non-directive. In particular, respondents are encouraged to describe events and perceptions in their own terms. The non-schedule standardised interview is especially suitable for collecting data that may have both 'objective' and 'subjective' elements. Examples of objective data would be the number of consultations the patients had with the doctor, and whether or not the patient received a prescription or advice about diet. Subjective data would include whether patients felt surprised, pleased or disappointed by a particular aspect of an outpatient visit. Subjective data can be obtained either from what people say or from the tone and manner with which it is said.

The data are tape-recorded. This is crucial for 'subjective' aspects of the interview. Such data can then be listened to and rated, in terms of simple rating scales, with considerable reliability. Tone and content of patients' accounts were taken into account in making ratings of the extent to which patients described their neurological clinic visits in positive, neutral or negative terms. Two dimensions of their visits emerged as salient and distinct. Patients had views about, on the one hand, the value of the medical treatment they received and, on the other hand, about the value of communication between themselves and the specialist. Although patients did describe and comment upon other aspects of their hospital visits, such as the length of time waiting for the appointment or time waiting at the clinic, these appeared to be of secondary importance overall.

## Expectations and concerns

Patients were asked about their expectations of the clinic visit before they saw the neurologist. Without exception patients were

uncertain and noncommittal in their replies. Few had received any
explanation from their general practitioner about the kind of specialist they were consulting, so only 44% knew that they were seeing
a neurologist. They therefore expressed only the vaguest guesses as
to what might happen at their outpatient appointment. These
guesses were informed by commonsense ideas of what normally
happens in medical consultations: the taking of a history, physical
examination, referral for some tests, and also by popular ideas of
the kinds of factors that might be medically relevant to the causes
of headaches, particularly diet and 'stress'. With regard to the outcomes of the visit, again patients went to great lengths to express
their uncertainty and the tentative nature of their hopes. The possibility of some explanation for symptoms, recommendations for
ways of avoiding episodes, and some kind of treatment were cited
by some respondents. However, repeatedly, patients emphasised
that they recognised the limitations of medical expertise and did
not expect 'miracle cures'. Others have commented on the mod-
esty of patients' expectations when seeking specialist care for
headache.[9,11]

If expectations were tentative, we were able to detect quite distinct concerns that patients had with regard to their symptoms. For
some patients, the main concern was distress and anxiety that their
headaches might be symptoms of a more serious underlying disease. This concern arose either because patients' symptoms had
persisted too long or had a significantly changed pattern such that
they could no longer be explained away as 'normal headaches'. A
number of patients' anxieties were increased by knowing personally someone with a medical problem such as a brain tumour or
haemorrhage. For this group of patients, a concern for *reassurance*
was a primary factor in seeking medical help.

A second and distinct group wanted an *explanation* for symptoms. Whilst not concerned about fears of brain tumours, they
were puzzled by a pattern of headaches that did not fit usual patterns. Different again were patients whose main concern was to
obtain some *preventive intervention*. The common factor in this
group related to what they did not want: they did not want further
symptomatic medical treatment. Many of this group had long-
standing histories of migraine and had received a variety of
symptomatic treatments from their general practitioner. Some of
the group hoped that a specialist might recommend preventive
medication; for others prevention would require advice about life-
style, diet, stress factors etc. Many of this group fitted Macintyre
and Oldman's description of the migraine patient as 'expert'.[12]

They had developed quite elaborate personal and experiential knowledge of their migraine in terms of provoking triggers, ameliorative actions, advantages and disadvantages of alternative therapies.

A final group of patients were concerned primarily to obtain *symptomatic relief*. As already argued, few expected something miraculous from the specialist; instead the view was that the neurologist was best placed to try 'something different' or 'something new'. Like other samples of chronic headache sufferers,[13] they had not experienced substantial benefits from either prescribed or non-prescribed medications, and they had no reason to expect anything different from the neurologist; he or she was more likely to be 'up to date' than their general practitioner.

## Satisfaction with the outpatient clinic

When patients were interviewed at home, we found a wide range of responses to the clinic visit, from very positive to very negative reactions. However, even patients who appeared very disappointed with the clinic were reluctant to describe themselves as 'dissatisfied'. Indeed often such respondents gave elaborate explanations of their reluctance to express negative views of the neurological consultation. Some were puzzled by aspects of the consultation. If the consultation appeared rushed or there had been no proper discussion of their symptoms, it was not clear whether it was because of their own behaviour or that of the doctor. In these circumstances, to be critical seemed inappropriate. For others this reluctance arose from a sense of sympathy or understanding for the constraints that prevail in the National Health Service (NHS); it would be unreasonable or inconsiderate to criticise. We were confronted by the normative beliefs that considerably inhibit the expression of critical attitudes regarding health care in the NHS and which must be one factor limiting the variability of questionnaire responses.[14,15] A common source of frustration for many patients in this study was what they felt to be a very rapid and controlling 'doctor centred' approach to history taking, which left the patient little time to express his concerns. However, when asked to summarise reactions to such experiences in terms of satisfaction, forgiving responses such as the following were typical: 'He [the consultant] was a very busy man. He made me so I couldn't think straight. You know there are other people outside. I know they can't help it. I sympathise.'

Although patients were reluctant to express attitudes in terms of

**Table 1.** Patient satisfaction with neurological consultation.

|  | Medical treatment | | Communication | |
|  | n | % | n | % |
|---|---|---|---|---|
| Positive (satisfied) | 37 | 39 | 29 | 31 |
| Neutral | 27 | 28 | 38 | 40 |
| Negative (dissatisfied) | 31 | 33 | 28 | 29 |
| *Total* | *95* | *100* | *95* | *100* |

dissatisfaction, their accounts of their hospital visits were striking for the range of negative as well as positive responses: at one extreme, for example, 'I must say I was very impressed. I don't know whether I was very lucky. I felt at last something was getting done' compared with, for example, 'I was disappointed and annoyed—a waste of time.' In both cases, it was as much the tone and manner of what was said as the content that revealed the first patient to have found the consultation successful, while the second judged it unsuccessful or disappointing.

Simple rating scales were used in relation to patients' views on the two most salient aspects of care—their reactions to their medical treatment and to the communication that occurred in the clinic visit. The results are shown in Table 1. For simplicity of presentation, patients are described as 'satisfied' or 'dissatisfied' although, as argued above, they themselves preferred not to use such attitudinal language to describe their views. The rating scales reflect the dominant tone of patients' comments; patients had to be quite critical to be rated as 'negative'. The following is part of an account by a patient rated as negative with regard to communication: 'He said I was physically OK and that the headaches would go as soon as they came but he would do an EEG to be sure. I was quite shocked, annoyed. My God, all he is saying is that they will go as soon as they came. How long do I have to wait? An absolute waste of time! I would have said: What are the causes of headaches like this? Instead I just sat there embarrassed. I got the impression he thought: Let's get this over and done with. He didn't ask me whether there was anything I wanted to ask. I was surprised he let me walk out without knowing anything.'

The content of the accounts by patients rated as negative were examined. Those who were negative about the medical content of their consultations were variously disappointed with: interpersonal aspects of the consultation (such as feeling that they had not been taken seriously); the limited history of their headaches taken by the doctor; lack or absence of investigations; the appropriateness or lack of treatment. Those who were negative about the communication aspects of their consultations mainly focused on the lack of any explanation for the diagnosis offered to them.[16]

### Explanations for dissatisfaction

A number of variables were found to be related to dissatisfaction. Patients with migraine, patients with longer histories of headache, and patients with a concern for preventive intervention were all significantly more likely than other patients to be dissatisfied with their consultations.[5] Close inspection of these cases showed that a group of patients with long-standing histories of migraine had developed quite complex views of the nature and causes of migraine. This group were particularly dissatisfied with what appeared to be a very superficial and limited investigation of their personal circumstances and life-style by the neurologist. Many felt that they had not been taken seriously and were disappointed that they had received no more attention than when they consulted their general practitioner. We viewed this as a mismatch between popular views that personalised advice about life-style could influence the course of headaches, the neurologist's more limited definition of his function, and knowledge of the poor scientific evidence for the efficacy of what is often written in popular books about migraine.

A second source of dissatisfaction could be traced to a different problem—failure to reassure. Most patients with concerns about brain tumours or other such possibilities were impressed with the specialist's reassurance. However, a minority remained very concerned about their symptoms after the hospital visit. They were dissatisfied with the explanations they had received. To some extent this may have been due to limitations in communication. The neurologist often failed to identify the presence of such worries.[16] Moreover, the reassurance that nothing is wrong is not effective if unsupported by substantive information.[17]

A third factor that proved to be significantly related to dissatisfaction was the presence of psychiatric symptoms. In some cases it appeared that dissatisfaction was part of a syndrome of unhappiness with the world in general.[18] For others it was more likely that the patient had insight into the inappropriateness of referral to the neurologist, given the limited psychosocial support role that he can play.

This brief explanation of the pattern of results has focused on the negative responses in the sample. It should be noted that many patients, particularly those wanting some alteration to their symptomatic treatment, and also the majority of those in need of reassurance, expressed positive satisfaction with the hospital visit.

One further result from the study should be briefly mentioned. It provides a curious form of construct validity for our measures of satisfaction. The sample of patients were followed up one year later, and a number of different assessments made of the changes to patients' headaches. We compared the severity of headaches as reported at the hospital visit with severity at one year follow-up, and also asked patients to rate the degree of change in symptoms. By either method, improvement in headaches was significantly associated with positive satisfaction one year previously.[19,20] Possible confounding effects such as severity of headache at consultation were ruled out. This result is very similar to that obtained in a Canadian study of patients presenting to their family doctors with headaches. The Headache Study Group found that the best outcomes after one year follow-up were in patients who felt they had been given sufficient opportunity to tell the doctor all they wanted to say at the initial visit.[21]

## Discussion

The approach to patient satisfaction described here is different from that found in most surveys. We examined intensively the experiences of patients who shared in common a single or at least a very similar health problem. This made it possible to get a clear focus on their perceptions of their problems and the benefits they obtained from medical care. Most important of all, we were able to integrate patients' perceptions of their problems with other relevant information, particularly the patient's health status and treatment. One of the most disappointing features of many patient satisfaction surveys is that they do not provide precise evidence of strengths and weaknesses of health care. Often the variation in satisfaction levels is explained by patients' demographic characteristics alone.[22] This means that patients' views in such studies are only minimally associated with aspects of quality of care. Although not providing a complete evaluation of the clinical setting which we were studying, patients' views produced invaluable qualitative and quantitative evidence of both positive and negative features of neurological management of headaches.

At the least this should demonstrate that patients' views have a place not only in managerial use of consumer surveys but also in medical audit. The patient can provide feedback that is relevant to core clinical activities. Moreover, we should also re-examine the range of subjects on which we seek to obtain patients' views. Patient satisfaction is least often measured with regard to outcomes.[23,24] This study indicates that the contribution of patients to assessment of health outcomes may be considerable.

Our approach to the recording and measurement of satisfaction is time-consuming and beyond the means of routine audit. It involves long interviews, with a strong emphasis on the patient's own concerns and agenda. Coding of such data requires the use of numerous rating scales that are sensitive to the tone and emphasis of recorded speech as much as the content. The methodology used was one primarily developed in social psychiatry where it has provided powerful and convincing explanations of social factors influencing the course of psychiatric illness.[25] In that field long-term work has enabled researchers to reduce and refine initially lengthy instruments without loss of sensitivity.[26] It may be possible to do the same thing with our in-depth approach to patient satisfaction. By comparison with other fields such as subjective health status measures, it is remarkable how little work has been done to assess the trades off between economy and sensitivity in the measurement of patient satisfaction. The main advantage associated with our methodology is that it enables close attention to be given to the varying concerns patients have regarding their health problems, and the varying extent to which concerns are resolved. This is a method that should be of particular interest in clinical applications of research into patient satisfaction.

## References

1. Pollitt C. Doing business in the temple? Managers and quality assurance in the public services. *Public Administration* 1990; **68**: 435–52.
2. Thomson R, Donaldson L. Medical audit and the wider quality debate. *Journal of Public Health Medicine* 1990; **12**: 149–51.
3. Reid M, Garcia J. Women's views of care during pregnancy and childbirth. In: Chalmers I, ed. *Effective care in pregnancy and childbirth.* Oxford: Oxford University Press, 1989: 131–42.
4. O'Brien B, Banner N, Gibson S, Yacoub M. The Nottingham Health Profile as a measure of quality of life following combined heart and lung transplantation. *Journal of Epidemiology and Community Health* 1988; **42**: 232–4.
5. Fitzpatrick R, Hopkins A. Illness behaviour and headache, and the sociology of consultations for headache. In: Hopkins A, ed. *Headache: problems in management.* London: W. Saunders, 1988: 351–5.

6. Grove J, Butler P, Millac P. The effect of a neurological clinic upon patients with tension headache. *Practitioner* 1980; **224**: 195–6.
7. Fitzpatrick R, Hopkins A. Referrals to neurologists for headaches not due to structural disease. *Journal of Neurology, Neurosurgery and Psychiatry* 1981; **44**: 1061–7.
8. Selby G, Lance J. Observations on 500 cases of migraine and allied vascular headache. *Journal of Neurology, Neurosurgery and Psychiatry* 1960; **23**: 23–33.
9. Packard R. What does the headache patient want? *Headache* 1979; **19**: 370–4.
10. Brown G, Rutter M. The measurement of family activities and relationships: a methodological study. *Human Relations* 1966; **19**: 241–63.
11. Edmeads J. Placebos and the power of negative thinking. *Headache* 1984; **24**: 342–3.
12. Macintyre S, Oldman D. Coping with migraine. In: Davis A, Horobin G, eds. *Medical encounters*. London: Croom Helm, 1977.
13. Parnell P, Cooperstock R. Tranquillisers and mood elevators in the treatment of migraine. *Headache* 1979; **19**: 78–89.
14. Locker D, Dunt D. Theoretical and methodological issues in sociological studies of consumer satisfaction with medical care. *Social Science and Medicine* 1978; **12**: 283–92.
15. Fitzpatrick R, Hopkins A. Problems in the conceptual framework of patient satisfaction research. *Sociology of Health and Illness* 1983; **5**: 297–311.
16. Fitzpatrick R, Hopkins A. Patients' satisfaction with communication in neurological outpatient clinics. *Journal of Psychosomatic Research* 1981; **25**: 329–34.
17. Kessell N. Reassurance. *Lancet* 1979; **i**: 1128–33.
18. Barsky A. Hidden reasons some patients visit doctors. *Annals of Internal Medicine* 1981; **94**: 492–8.
19. Fitzpatrick R, Hopkins A. Effects of referral to a specialist for headache. *Journal of the Royal Society of Medicine* 1983; **76**: 112–5.
20. Fitzpatrick R, Hopkins A, Harvard-Watts O. Social dimensions of healing: a longitudinal study of outcomes of medical management of headaches. *Social Science and Medicine* 1983; **17**: 501–10.
21. Headache Study Group. Predictors of outcome in headache patients presenting to family physicians. *Headache* 1986; **26**: 285–94.
22. Fitzpatrick R. Measurement of patient satisfaction. In: Hopkins A, Costain D, eds. *Measuring the outcomes of medical care*. London: Royal College of Physicians and King's Fund Centre, 1990.
23. Hall J, Dornan M. Meta-analysis of satisfaction with medical care: description of research domain and analysis of overall satisfaction levels. *Social Science and Medicine* 1988; **27**: 637–44.
24. Cleary P, McNeil B. Patient satisfaction as an indicator of quality of care. *Inquiry* 1988; **25**: 25–36.
25. Brown G, Harris T. *The social origins of depression*. London: Tavistock, 1978.
26. Vaughn C, Leff J. The influence of family and social factors in the course of psychiatric illness. *British Journal of Psychiatry* 1976; **129**: 125–37.

# 7 | Critical incident technique as a method of assessing patient satisfaction

**Michael Pryce-Jones**
*The Oxford Consultancy, Oxford*

Critical incident technique is a qualitative method of enquiry designed to identify causes of satisfaction and dissatisfaction from interviewing patients. Most patient satisfaction surveys are quantitative and use methods based on market research or opinion polling; they produce numerical statements of opinions held on a range of topics but often cannot give any precise indication of why the opinions were formed. Critical incident technique, on the other hand, pinpoints the causes that underlie value judgements and is not concerned primarily with numbers of opinions held.

All enquiry methods to patients have inherent flaws[1] but it can be argued that critical incident technique avoids many of the difficulties commonly associated with conventional methods. However, it is no exception to the general principle and is itself prone to objections not found in quantitative approaches.

The technique was first employed by the United States Army Air Force during the closing years of World War 2 to improve unit combat efficiency. It was later used in industrial training and management applications in North America. It appears to have been established academically by John Flanagan in 1954.[2]

The Industrial Training Unit in association with North West Thames Regional Health Authority were probably the first to use it in the UK specifically for patient enquiries.[3] Since then the method has been developed and used effectively in Oxford, mostly to evaluate the quality of service in outpatient departments[4] but also with surgical inpatients, discharged elderly patients (to test discharge procedures) and in general practice.[5]

## Critical incident theory

The theory is based on the premise that feelings of satisfaction or dissatisfaction stem mainly from events experienced by the subject

which cause him or her to form value judgements. Thus any
episode of experience is composed of a series of events, some of
which may cause good feelings, some bad, and some neither good
nor bad. An incident is critical only if it triggers a value judgement;
otherwise it is neutral and of no interest. This point can be illustrated by three comments:

> 'The receptionist smiled at me and addressed me by name'
> [good]
> 'She repeated my personal details in a loud voice that everyone
> could hear' [bad]
> 'She wrote everything down with her left hand' [neutral]

If good and bad incidents can be identified, the good ones can be
made to happen more often, the bad ones eliminated or modified,
and thus the level of patient satisfaction raised. For instance, from
the episode above, receptionists could be trained always to smile,
address patients by name, and never repeat personal details in
such a way as to be overheard by others.

In the context of assessing patient satisfaction, it has been helpful in interviewer training to define the range of critical incidents
that might be encountered during enquiries. These broad categories are:

(a) Any action or inaction that causes an opinion to be formed
(b) Any action or inaction governed by a procedure or mode of
behaviour that causes an opinion to be formed
(c) An environmental or other factor the presence or absence of
which causes an opinion to be formed

The first two categories are not mutually exclusive but it can be
helpful to make a distinction when the data are used to make
changes in the design of training programmes, in procedures or in
staff attitudes. For example, a discretionary one-off action on the
part of an individual can be compared with an incident arising
from the imposition of a procedure, eg a block appointment system. There is a difference between an inaction when a published
procedure was not followed and one when no action was taken
when an action was desirable although not prescribed, eg a patient
not told about a delay in appointments. The remedies in each case
would be different.

Actions or inactions, when they stem solely from the exercise of
clinical judgement, have been excluded from the range of
enquiries carried out up to now.

As regards environmental factors, within the critical incident theory, these may be viewed as the effects of actions or inactions in the past. A common example is the failure of Health Authorities to provide adequate car parking space near an outpatient department (inaction in the past).

Some examples from outpatient department studies illustrate these definitions:

(a) Action/inaction

'When I came here on my own, the nurses came and had a chat with me. If you are feeling lonely and a bit low that is very nice.'

'I had to wait for nearly 2 hours; nobody told me why. If I had not spent the money on a taxi I would have gone without seeing the doctor.'

(b) Procedure/behaviour mode

'It is ridiculous. Everybody has got an appointment for 10.30. There must be about 20 of us here with only one doctor.'

'The doctor introduced herself and explained the diagnosis and what she was going to do, and when she was doing it she explained what was happening at every stage.'

(c) Environmental

'The pictures and plants in the waiting area cheer the place up if you have to wait a bit.'

'There's only one loo and when there are lots of people it's not really enough.'

Other ways of defining the types and range of critical incidents may be devised for specific enquiries, but for general purposes in the training context these definitions have been found adequate.

**The technique**

In brief, critical incident technique involves trained interviewers talking to patients individually, in private and in confidence. Patients are encouraged to talk freely to the interviewer and to recount any incident that they consider important and that led them to form good or bad views about the service. Open questions are used to elicit a response. Critical incidents are recorded manually on a semi-structured questionnaire. There are three necessary conditions. In order to capture critical incidents successfully:

- Patients must be convinced that the enquiry is entirely confidential and that what they say is non-attributable.

- Patients must not be led during the interview but allowed to say freely what impressed them favourably or unfavourably.
- Interviewers must be properly trained to relate professionally to the subjects and to be able to recognise and record critical incidents.

These conditions can be met as described below.


*Confidentiality*

Measures to guarantee confidentiality vary with the object of the enquiry but in all cases the interviewers must be seen to be independent of the service being reviewed. It is not reasonable to expect patients who might need further care from the same source to speak frankly about their experiences to someone closely associated with providing their present care.

In the contexts of general practice, outpatient and accident and emergency departments, where large numbers of patients are available and the population is constantly changing, written notices are handed to each patient on arrival at the reception point and distributed in the waiting area. The text explains briefly the nature of the survey and stresses that the interviewer will not ask the patient's name, that many patients will be interviewed and that it is the patient's experiences that are of interest, not his or her identity. It is also made clear that there is no obligation at all on the patient to participate.

Patients are approached by interviewers, after completing their consultation or treatment, and asked if they will take part in the study. If they agree, they are taken to a nearby room and at the onset the interviewer again emphasises that what is said is entirely unattributable.

Sometimes it is necessary to visit patients at their homes, for example in the case of patients who have been discharged from hospital, or housebound patients in general practice surveys. On these occasions, the names and addresses of the subjects must clearly be known to the interviewers, so assurances of confidentiality cannot be presented quite so cogently. The essential points conveyed to patients are that the interviewers are independent of the ward, department, service or practice, and that there is no obligation on anyone to take part. On occasions it may be necessary when preparing a report to omit either completely or partially elements in the critical incident which might identify a patient.

*Conduct of interviews*

The rationale of the interview requires that the subject should feel relaxed and be able to speak freely to the interviewer, unconstrained by formality or anxiety. Interviewers are trained to use various devices to achieve these ends. The environment for the interviews is also important. Clinical rooms should be avoided; preferable are rooms with informal furnishings as opposed to desks and office furniture. Central to the philosophy of the critical incident technique is that interviews should focus on the patient's agenda and not on that of the interviewer. Yet, at the same time, there is a need for some structure within which that agenda can be contained. It is also necessary that the events seen by the patient as critical be recorded as far as possible in the patient's own words. These aims are achieved by using a specially designed semi-structured questionnaire; this document separates the episodes of the experience under review into sequential or generic stages which can be represented by a page. For example, in a general practice study, the first stage might be 'Making the appointment', the next 'Getting to the surgery', the next 'Reception arrangements', and so on. Patients are asked about their experiences initially by open questions, eg 'How did you feel about . . .?', to elicit a response. Secondary questions or prompts can be used at the interviewer's discretion to probe areas partially exposed by a general expression of like or dislike. Prompts are also generally framed as open questions. It is stressed in the training programmes for interviewers that the cardinal error is to lead.

Interviewers need not follow the sequence of the questionnaire, and often may leave out entire stages if the patient expresses no interest in them. Having encouraged subjects to talk freely, the interviewers record the key words and phrases used to describe the critical events. After the conclusion of the interview they write out, as near to verbatim as possible, the critical incidents in the appropriate part of the questionnaire.

*Training of interviewers*

Any enquiry using critical incident technique relies on the effectiveness of the interviewers, who have a great deal of discretion in the way they encourage patients to relate their experiences. The selection of potential interviewers is of prime importance. Ideally they should be mature personalities with sufficient knowledge of the service to enable them to recognise the significance of what

the patients say, and with personal qualities that enable them both
to inspire the patients to talk freely and to refrain from leading
those interviewed or influencing what they say in any way. Interviewers may be employed by an organisation independent of the
unit whose services are being reviewed (such as a consultancy
firm), or they may be employees of the unit who are released from
their normal duties to interview on a part-time basis. If they are of
the latter category, as has already been stressed, it is vital that
members of staff selected have no connection with the part of the
service being studied. This is because the integrity of the technique may be compromised if interviewers are seen by patients
and departmental staff as part of the service for which the
information is being sought.

Provided the selection criteria are met, interviewers can be
trained in a relatively short time. Elements in the training consist
of the theory of critical incident technique and the practical skills
of identifying, capturing and recording critical incidents. Special
emphasis is placed on the initial approach to patients, and on ways
in which they can be encouraged to speak freely and spontan-
eously about their experiences. The phrasing of open questions,
the recognition of coded responses which require further explanation, and the need to probe value judgements figure prominently
in this part of the training. At the end of this, trainees should have
sufficient knowledge of the theory and practice to be able to conduct interviews adequately and without supervision. However, as
with all skills, effectiveness improves with practice. Experience suggests that a properly trained and experienced interviewer might be
expected to carry out five or six interviews of outpatients in the
course of a half-day session.

## Presentation of the results

At the end of any enquiry, individual interviewers will have collected a substantial number of critical incidents. It will then be necessary for the survey manager to present the results in a way in which
they can be used most effectively to improve the quality of the service. The way in which the results are presented will therefore
depend on the purpose for which the survey was designed. In
studies of outpatient, accident and emergency and general practice, it has been found helpful to group the critical incidents in a
way that reflects the sequence of events and follows patients
through the system. In a study of discharged inpatients, the critical
incidents were grouped to mirror the elements in the procedure,

**Table 1.** Summary of critical incidents.

| Stage | Favourable | Unfavourable | Total |
|---|---|---|---|
| Making the appointment | 10 | 11 | 21 |
| Getting to and from outpatients | 11 | 26 | 37 |
| Reception/waiting area and diagnostic departments | 38 | 49 | 87 |
| Consultation/treatment | 25 | 15 | 40 |
| *Total* | *84* | *101* | *185* |

for example advice about medicines, home equipment, arrangements for the follow-up and so on, so that the strengths and weaknesses of current practice were illustrated.

Although the technique is entirely qualitative, it can be useful to present a numerical summary of critical incidents, showing the number of favourable and unfavourable incidents identified in each category; this both illustrates the categories and the balance in numerical terms between favourable and unfavourable incidents. Such a summary effectively outlines the contents of the qualitative text, even though it has no significance on its own. Table 1 shows a typical numerical summary of critical incidents taken from an outpatient study.

As the enquiry is qualitative, not quantitative, the number of patients interviewed is not statistically determined. A sample is obtained that is broadly representative of the population in receipt of the service being surveyed. In outpatients some determinants of satisfaction will be the same for all specialties; others may relate to certain specialties only. Similarly, in general practice it is important to interview patients who have been in contact with health visitors and practice community nurses as well as those whose dealings have been only with their doctors.

The textual element of the report is in the form of an inventory of critical incidents. The way in which they are presented has already been discussed but there remains the question of what should or should not be included. There are some general principles. On receipt of the completed questionnaires, editors should ensure that each entry is indeed a critical incident, as inexperienced interviewers may occasionally mistake elaborate value judgements for critical incidents, and that ambiguous incidents, for example 'They always call you by your first name', must be clearly labelled favourable or unfavourable according to the perception of the subject. If an incident is so specific that there is a chance that the patient could be identified, the editor will need to decide how best to present the incident to preserve confidentiality.

The inclusion of every critical incident in the inventory has the merit of allowing the reader to see the entire range of incidents collected. In smaller scale studies there may be advantages in this. However, when several hundred incidents are recorded and many make the same point, it is usually best to produce illustrative examples rather than to include every item in the inventory which can then become repetitive and tedious to read. Although numbers of similar statements often have value in indicating good and bad points in the service provided, it must be remembered that a single critical incident may be highly significant in qualitative value.

## Putting the results into use

When the study is complete and the report and inventory have been published, there are a variety of ways in which the material may be used. Critical incidents have been found to be especially useful as catalytic agents in quality circles or quality improvement groups. This is because all the incidents are directly relevant to the service under review. As the inventory shows favourable as well as unfavourable opinion-forming events, staff do not feel threatened. The 'good' practices are clearly identified and can be built upon to improve the service.

The critical incidents can be used for the agreement and establishment of quality standards. For example, in an outpatient study, several incidents relating to the cancellation of appointments and the reallocation of appointments were discovered. All were unfavourable for different reasons. This led to the development of a quality standard which provided that, in the event of the cancellation of an appointment, apologies were to be given, patients were to be offered a choice of a new appointment time and, as a general principle, no patient was to have an appointment cancelled more than once.

If the collected critical incidents are not used in specific quality applications, they can be a powerful agent for procedural change. They provide direct and unbiased data from the people or departments affected by procedures or lack of procedures. For example, it was discovered in one outpatient survey that every patient attending was asked on the appointment form to bring a urine sample. Many patients ignored this request, but for those who did as they were asked there were no clear procedures for acceptance of the sample, and in some cases patients were told that it was not necessary for them to have brought one. The clear indications were to change the practice for obtaining samples, and to establish a procedure for their receipt and processing in the department.

Finally, because of their even-handed and direct nature, critical incidents can be used effectively in staff training programmes, determining some of the content of training and providing examples of the effects of types of behaviour on patients.

## Advantages of the method

Critical incident technique overcomes a number of the criticisms to which conventional methods of data collection are commonly subject. Some of these are described below.

### Designer bias

Designers of questionnaires generally cover topics that they feel are important, but these are not necessarily what the patient thinks important. Critical incident technique allows the patient to choose the agenda.

### Effects not causes

Quantitative methods are designed to produce numerical state-ments of effects (numbers of opinions held) without identifying primary causes. Critical incident technique pinpoints individual causes of satisfaction and dissatisfaction and enables them to be addressed immediately.

### Diminution of minority views

If an opinion is held only by a relatively small number of people, in numerical terms this appears to be a relatively insignificant prob-lem. However, in qualitative terms the problem may be highly sig-nificant. Critical incident technique gives equal weight to each incident discovered.

### Inhibition

Patients may be reluctant to criticise an organisation from which they are receiving treatment, because they are anxious that it might adversely affect their treatment in the future,[6] or they may believe that to criticise any aspect of the service that helped to make them feel better is ungrateful.[7] Critical incident technique does not disclose the identity of the patient. Since 'good' incidents as well as 'bad' incidents are obtained, patients do not feel ungrateful in criticising those aspects of service that annoyed them, because they can praise others that they thought were particularly well performed.

*Inconvenience*

Some subjects do not like filling in questionnaires, and others may have a problem with language or literacy. Critical incident technique interviewers are trained to make the interview a pleasant and sociable occasion. In addition, there is no compulsion on patients to participate; indeed it is made easy for them to refuse.

The main strength of the method lies in its directness: from the inventory of critical incidents, patients speak directly to the providers of the service. The information is recognised as being authentic and immediately useful. Furthermore, because of the even-handed presentation of 'good' or 'bad' events, staff do not feel threatened. Reports have been found to be excellent catalytic material in quality circles and quality improvement groups, as well as providing a basis for managers to change procedures, design training programmes or make environmental improvements.

## Disadvantages of the method

*Statistical reservations*

One of the objections made against critical incident technique is that it is statistically unsound, unlike quantitative surveys which have statistically based sample sizes. It cannot be denied that this is the case, but there is a distinction between quantitative and qualitative methods, and a distinction between statistical and practical significance. The technique is not suited to wider generalised enquiries which measure and monitor levels of patient satisfaction. It is more appropriate to localised applications where the specific qualitative data can be related to a department, a service, or a specialty.

*Sectional over-representation*

As interviews are entirely voluntary, critical incident technique may over-represent patients who are articulate and sociable, to the detriment of the reticent or shy.

*Demanding of labour and skill*

Critical incident technique relies on the skill of the interviewers, who need to be specially trained. Although the training itself can be carried out effectively in a day (the usual procedure is to train Health Authority staff locally), it is important to select people who have the requisite knowledge of the service and whose personality enables them easily to relate to strangers. Thus it can be more skill intensive than most conventional enquiries. If it is necessary to visit patients at home, as in the case of discharged patients, it can also be labour intensive.

## Summary

Critical incident technique is equipped to provide a range and depth of information not available from other methods of measuring patient satisfaction. The specific nature of the data allows an immediate response to causes of satisfaction and dissatisfaction. However, it is not suited to quantitative measurement in its wider sense. It is probably more labour and skill intensive than most quantitative techniques, but not necessarily more expensive in producing results of value to the service and to future patients.

## References

1.  Pryce-Jones M, Learmonth M, Totterdell B. Using customer satisfaction surveys to improve service quality. *Health Services Management* 1990; **86**: 273–4.
2.  Flanagan JC. The critical incident technique. *Psychological Bulletin* 1954; **5**: 327–58.
3.  Callaghan D, Caple T. *Managing customer relations*. London: North West Thames Regional Health Authority and Industrial Training Unit, 1986.
4.  Pryce-Jones DM. Not how many but why: a qualitative approach to customer relations. *Health Services Management* 1986; **84**: 175–7.
5.  Gau D, Pryce-Jones M, Tippins D. Satisfactory practice. *Health Service Journal* 1989; 30 November: 1464–5.
6.  Hurst K, Ball J. Service with a smile. *Health Service Journal* 1990; 25 January: 120–1.
7.  Greenley JR, Schulz R, Sung Hee Nam, Peterson RW. Patient satisfaction with psychiatric inpatient care. *Research in Community and Mental Health* 1987; **5**: 307–19.

# 8 | The doctor's perspective

**Anthony Hopkins**
*Research Unit, Royal College of Physicians, London*

The first duty of physicians must be to make their patients 'feel better'. This applies whether the physician is reassuring a patient with a tension headache, or helping a patient come to terms with irremediable malignant disease. Satisfaction with a physician's services—literally that he or she has 'done enough'—is therefore a most important outcome of medical care. Delivery of skilled technical procedures, such as the relief of acute urinary retention by catheterisation, understandably results in a satisfied patient, because of the acute relief of unpleasant and continuing symptoms. However, the usual ready control of acute infections by antibiotics has meant that, for the present generation of doctors, the accent of medical care is on the management of chronic disorders and the maintenance of health in older age. Patient satisfaction therefore assumes increasing dominance as a dimension of outcome of any intervention. A proper subject for research, therefore, is to examine how interventions can be carried out in such a way that more satisfaction is produced, in exactly the same way as other research is carried out to determine how longer remissions can be induced in cancer, or strokes more certainly prevented by carotid endarterectomy.

Just as technical outcomes of care are often multidimensional (avoidance of mortality, avoidance of recurrence, avoidance of wound infection, relief of pain, and so on), so is the outcome of satisfaction with care. For example, a woman may be well pleased with a surgical scar and the relief of intestinal colic resulting from a successful operation on a chronic intestinal obstruction. However, she may have been less pleased with the time she had to wait for her operation, the surgeon's attitude towards her, the amount of information she was given about the nature of her illness, the continuity of nursing care that she received, and so on.

Clinicians perceive much of the literature about patient satisfaction to be weak insofar as it fails to reflect what they regard as important aspects of medical care. Many patient satisfaction questionnaires (see Chapter 5) concentrate upon aspects of care that are comparatively easy to monitor, such as satisfaction with waiting times. This is largely because the attribute (eg time waiting in out-patients) can be readily measured, and the patient's satisfaction with this time can also be readily measured on a Likert scale. Some physicians and surgeons have formerly taken the robust attitude that it may not matter too much how long the patient waits, as long as the technical care and the technical outcome of the procedure are good. However, there is increasing realisation that the profes-sional and ethical constraints within which doctors operate are such that they and patients should enter an equal partnership in solving a patient's problems, and in such partnerships proper respect should be paid to patients' values, including the time that they spend waiting, and their loss of income if they are sent for an operation that is then cancelled. Furthermore, although satisfac-tion with care is a measure of outcome of that care, it can also influence future health status. For example, a patient who has been very dissatisfied with a procedure is less likely to return for appropriate follow-up and possible further effective interventions.

It follows therefore that physicians need to know the principal attributes of health care that should be reflected in any considera-tion of satisfaction. Without dissecting out the various dimensions of care with which patients can be satisfied or dissatisfied, it is diffi-cult to see how individual changes can be made to increase patient satisfaction. Table 1 presents one way in which a physician can organise his thoughts about patient satisfaction with care.

## Satisfaction with the availability of care

Richardson and colleagues[1] have recently explored the health ser-vices thought to be important by a random sample of the popula-tion of Bath, in the UK. Of the ten services proposed to respond-ents, renal dialysis and special care baby units were thought most frequently to be very important. The larger scale surveys of public opinion in Oregon are well known (eg reference 2). A mismatch between the services thought to be important by the population and those provided could be used as a measure of population satis-faction.

The availability of care in the sense of providing suitable num-bers of trained personnel and appropriately sited hospitals and modern and effective equipment and services therein is a matter for central government and their designated health authorities. However, an individual physician has a responsibility to the health care system in which he works to bring to the attention of his

**Table 1**. Some dimensions of satisfaction with care.

---

Availability of care,
   eg Are there suitably trained physicians?
       Do resource constraints limit care?

Accessibility of care,
   eg Time waiting for care
       Affordability of care
       Distance to travel for care

Process of care,
   eg Technical competence
       Interpersonal aspects of care:
           Continuity of care
           Time spent by doctors with patients
           Empathy of doctors with patients
           Providing information
       Organisation of care

Outcomes of care,
   eg Relief of pain
       Cure of disease
       Restoration of function
       Cosmetic improvement

---

See also Table 1 in Chapter 1.

health authority through its Medical Advisory Committee structure obvious deficiencies in the structure of care. If, for example, an intervention known to be effective is not delivered to the local population, it is right that physicians who know the procedure to be effective should press for the institution of that intervention. This is an important point, as patients may be satisfiled with relatively low levels of care, through ignorance. If they knew of the local unavailability of interventions known to be effective, then they might well become dissatisfied. It is, incidentally, a concern among many specialist groups that the purchaser/provider split instituted by the NHS and Community Care Act of 1990 has led to fragmentation of the previous moderately efficient Regional Medical Advisory Committee structure.

Although the rational allocation of resources (rationing) is largely outside the province of the individual physician at the macro-economic level, this is not so at the micro-economic level. A hospital consultant in charge of a busy department may be responsible for the disbursement in salary and other costs of several million pounds each year. Increasingly, physicians are asked to work within budgets, and just like anyone else in charge of a budget they have to decide what they can and cannot afford to do. There are ethical issues here that have not yet been generally ventilated; this is rationing within a directorate for budgetary reasons. Until the early 1980s physicians or surgeons would be as busy as they could be, putting in pacemakers and using expensive chemotherapeutic drugs, because they believed that that was what they were paid to do. In general, they did not consider that by doing so they might be distorting the provision of care in the hospital by limiting funds for other specialties. The advent of clinical directorates has largely prevented that. Now a cardiologist will, for example, have to decide to put in a pacemaker that is technically inferior to one he or she knows could do a better job but which is considerably more expensive. At present, patients are unlikely to be aware of such technical issues, but they certainly are aware of constrained resources if they request a head scan and are informed that their clinical need is not sufficient to allow the budgetary disbursement. On the whole, physicians and surgeons are only just beginning to have to face patients dissatisfied on these grounds. There is, however, one exception in which dissatisfaction is very rapidly growing, and that is the institution from 1 April 1993 of the purchasing of packages of health care for disabled and elderly people in the community by local directorates of social services. At present, a frail elderly person may have free hospital care in a long-stay geriatric ward. However, such an elderly person, on moving into the community, may have to contribute financially to the packages of care put together by the directorates of social services. Some families are already making their dissatisfaction known at the way the savings of a lifetime can rapidly be expended in purchasing care for an elderly relative.

## Satisfaction with access to care

The example just cited illustrates the border between availability and accessibility. The non-availability of free NHS geriatric beds means that some other types of long-term care are accessible only to those relatives with sufficiently deep pockets. Geographical accessibility is another aspect that may lead to patient dissatisfaction. For example, the allocation of resources may mean that a Regional Health Authority decides to concentrate the provision of a specialised technical intervention, such as radiotherapy, in one or two sites which are remote from large numbers of the Regional population. The local population may prefer to have locally accessible care even if it is technically slightly inferior to that which is far distant. People receiving radiotherapy for cancer, for example, may value easy access for themselves and for their relatives to visit rather than the latest high-tech care which achieves only marginal gains in outcome. There may be therefore a trade off between accessibility and technical competence, and it is likely that some patients will be dissatisfied with either one or the other.

Then there is availability of time. Here again there are trades off. In general, people like to spend a long time with their doctors, in order to ensure that the doctor fully understands the situation that is affecting their lives, and so that the doctor can explain fully what he or she proposes. However, the longer a doctor spends with one patient, the longer he or she will keep another waiting. The institution of the *Patient's Charter*,[3] with the entirely praiseworthy object of laying down times in outpatients beyond which patients should not have to wait, does not recognise that this is in conflict with the time spent with other patients in explaining the nature of their illness. One thing that impresses all physicians is how busy they are. It may well be that a more focused organisation of time would make more time available for direct clinical contact, but physicians generally feel that these conflicts are inadequately recognised.

## Satisfaction with the process of care

I illustrate this aspect of patient satisfaction using the traditional consultation, often in outpatients—what our fellow health service researchers in the United States often call an 'ambulatory encounter'. All that goes on within a consultation, and which may result in satisfaction or dissatisfaction, can be broadly conceptualised in two dimensions. In the instrumental task of the consultation, the patient and physician both give information and ask questions, and the physician undertakes technical procedures; in the socio-emotional dimension, the two (or more) protagonists build partnerships, often partly by conversation and acts such as social conversation which are not directly related to the instrumental tasks of care.[4]

### *Instrumental task-orientated aspects of medical care: technical competence*

The first issue concerns patients' ability to tell whether their doctor is technically competent. There are certain areas in which it is difficult if not impossible for a patient to have much idea about this. For example, competence in fine apposition of small blood vessels is a necessary prerequisite for a successful outcome in coronary bypass surgery, but a patient with coronary artery disease, anaesthetised, can have no idea about how well this technical task is being performed. Yet the patient has indirect channels—the 'reputation' of the physician or surgeon. Although difficult to quantify, informal networks of information do seem to inform general practitioners about surgeons who have successful results, and others who have more adverse outcomes. The outcome of these informal networks may, in some health care systems, be a large private practice. However, interpersonal aspects of care probably play a substantial part in building up a successful practice, and are probably more important than poorly informed views about technical outcomes.

The competence in suturing a coronary artery is an extreme example, as many technical procedures, particularly when carried out by physicians as opposed to surgeons, are not open to the patient's inspection. One might postulate that even an educated but lay patient would have little information on which to base an assessment of the competence of, for example, an examination of the cardiovascular or neurological systems. However, possibly informed in this age by television and movies, patients do seem to have a moderately well informed idea of what should be done. For example, Davies and Ware[5] and Chang and colleagues (cited in reference 5) have video-recorded six simulated provider–patient encounters that deliberately manipulated three aspects of care (technical, psycho-social, patient participation) for a repeat outpatient consultation for previously diagnosed angina. The quality of the technical aspects of care was rated by physicians, and lay people then rated the tapes. Interviews that were scripted to include necessary and sufficient history and items of physical examination were rated by participants significantly more favourably than low technical quality consultations that omitted relevant and included irrelevant items.

These results were obtained in the United States, and it is possible that in a less informed constituency people may be less able to rate the technical aspects of care. In our study on tension headaches, described in Chapter 6, patients with tension headaches interviewed before their consultations with a neurologist had very vague and ill-formed ideas of what to expect. However, once in the consultation, their expectations did seem to crystallise, and a few patients were dissatisfied with technical aspects of care, namely what the neurologist did, though many more were dissatisfied with communication and other interpersonal aspects.[6,7]

There is some evidence that at least some patients equate technical quality with quantity of care. Davies and Ware[5] suggest that the proponents of this argument hold that consumers can be 'seduced by the kind or number of tests and procedures received into believing that services provided were appropriate and well performed'. Sox and his colleagues studied men with chest pain of a type considered on the basis of a clinical algorithm not to require tests to rule out a myocardial infarction. However, patients who were randomly assigned to have an electrocardiogram and to have their serum levels of creatine phosphokinase measured, which is elevated if there has truly been a myocardial infarction, evaluated their overall care more favourably than did those who had not undergone the investigations.[8] Again, however, such observations are not generalisable to all clinical situations. In my study with Fitzpatrick on tension headaches, we found no significant relationship between patient satisfaction and the investigations performed.[6,7] We do not know how stable such observations are. Our research was carried out in the early days of brain scanning. The same results in this clinical situation might well not be found if the study were repeated now.

Both the studies cited related to clinical situations in which there were no adverse clinical outcomes.[6–8] I know of no systematic study of how people view adverse outcomes. Clinical experience indicates a range of opinion from extreme dissatisfaction (for example, with unexpected severe incontinence after transurethral prostatectomy) through resignation along the lines of 'I am sure he did his best, and he tells me the operation proved unexpectedly difficult'. Extreme dissatisfaction with outcomes of technical procedures can of course spill over into complaints and even litigation for malpractice. It is here that risk management has its place—the identification of risks within a system of care and a pro-active attempt to remove or minimise the risks.

Patients may also express dissatisfaction with the technical aspects of care by silently or openly failing to comply with medical advice. For example, a man prescribed a beta-blocking drug to lower his blood pressure may fail to take the tablets, not because of any failure in communication, but because adverse outcomes of mild depression and impaired potency are such that, as far as he is concerned, the technical intervention is just not worthwhile. In such an instance, patients are well able to make their own judgements about the value of the intervention, although they may be less than adequately informed about the risks that they are running if they do not follow the suggested treatment plan.

Patients have other ways of gaining information about the technical quality of care that they may expect. This may be through informal channels such as the experience of relatives or friends, or more formal channels such as the register of medical specialists maintained by the General Medical Council in this country, or by the specialty boards in the United States. It is expected that technical competence is likely to be greater if appropriate training has been recognised by accreditation or by registration or board-certification as a specialist.[9]

### Socio-emotional aspects of care

*Humane care.* In a meta-analysis of the literature on patient satisfaction, Hall and Dornan found that 'humaneness' ranked second only to 'overall quality' in importance.[10] I draw attention briefly to some particular aspects of this most important aspect of care.

Roter and Hall have reviewed the available literature on doctor–patient interaction, and provide a useful framework for its consideration.[11] The dimensions they identify include the exchange of information including counselling and advice, the desirability of concordance between patient and physician on what the problems are, conveyed affect, and patient confidence. Much of the research in this field depends upon the analysis of tape-recorded or video-recorded consultations, so it is not suitable for routine use in measuring patient satisfaction. However, post-consultation interviews are a powerful tool at understanding the patient perspectives of the consultation. In Chapter 6, Fitzpatrick and I review our earlier work on patients with headache, and draw particular attention to the ill-formed nature of the patient's expectations before consultation, the concern for information and reassurance, and the concern for prevention and for symptomatic relief. In our studies (reviewed also in references 6, 7 and 12), as in others, patients were dissatisfied if they perceived that the doctor treated the consultation as 'routine', without recognising the individuality of the problem to the patient. There was also considerable dissatisfaction related to explanation of the diagnosis and the implications for the future.

There are numerous studies (see reference 11 for further references) on the importance of the doctor's affect on patient satisfaction. An uninterested doctor, even if technically competent, will have many dissatisfied patients.

*Continuity of care.* In a busy metropolitan life, continuity of environment and small relationships with that environment do clearly pro-

vide a sense of identity and well-being.[13] It is not surprising therefore that patients like to see the same doctor on repeated visits,
because they are aware that the doctor knows about their social
background and previous illness which may well influence any
interventions that are proposed. Hjortdahl and Laerum suggest
that the patient's expectations are again important: '. . . with continuity of care and accumulated knowledge about the specific physician and the consultation setting, the patient's standard may be set
more realistically, and major discrepancies between expectation
and experience may be less common, thus increasing the likeli-
hood of satisfaction. Furthermore, the personal relations that frequently develop in an ongoing patient–doctor relationship may
increase patients' tolerance by widening the latitudes of acceptance around their subjective standard, thereby increasing the
chance of satisfaction'.[14] These authors showed that, if a patient
considered the doctor he attended for a consultation to be his personal doctor for all his health problems, the odds ratio of the
patient being satisfied compared with a situation in which the consultation was not with his 'personal doctor' was nearly sevenfold.

Continuity of care not only leads to increased satisfaction with a
consultation; satisfaction ratings can be used to predict what
patients will do when they next need health services.[15] In the United States, disenrolment from a community health care plan is
taken as one measure of dissatisfaction with a planned service, and
leavers will often receive a questionnaire asking them what was
wrong. Although, in many instances, disenrolment resulted from a
misunderstanding of the terms of membership of the health plan,
some members left because of perceived poor professional competence and the unwillingness of the staff to discuss their problems.[16]
Table 3 on page 72 also illustrates that in the UK those who change
their general practitioner (without changing their address) are less
likely to be satisfied with their care. Those who change general
practitioners may of course do so until they find a doctor fitting
their own style and expectations. This in part may be associated
with the significant increase in satisfaction found with long-standing personal care.[14]

The evidence seems overwhelming that continuity of care is
highly valued by patients, but again the bind in which physicians
find themselves is, I believe, not adequately recognised. Family
doctors and hospital registrars both need time off, and the pressure to reduce junior doctors' hours is going to have a substantial
impact on continuity of care in hospital wards. Although the recognition of the importance of the continuity of nursing care means

that most patients are now assigned a primary nurse, the pressures on staff are such that a patient may see little more of his or her primary nurse than of any other nurse; in those hospitals now operating a shift system for junior staff, the patient may be looked after by three different young doctors in the space of twenty-four hours. Here is another example in which the research evidence of what is satisfactory care and the pressures of resource constraint are in direct conflict.

*Organisational aspects of care*

There are some non-medical aspects of the process of care for which patients may rightly be dissatisfied with doctors, noteworthy amongst these being prolonged waits in outpatient clinics due to poor planning of the clinic, which must be under a consultant's control. In other ways, too, poor management structures within a hospital may reflect upon a patient's satisfaction with the consultation itself. For example, if the medical records department fails to find the medical records from the previous consultation, or the results of an investigation, it is not likely that the patient will be satisfied with the outcome of the consultation. In these circumstances the doctor, perhaps justifiably irritated by the absence of administrative support, may be unjustifiably short and abrupt with his patient.

**Outcomes of care**

The first sentence of this chapter recorded that the first duty of physicians must be to make their patients 'feel better'. By better, we mean an improvement in health status, including psychological and cognitive components of health status, and health-related quality of life.[17] Until recently, health services have been driven by measures of activity (discharges and deaths per available bed, for example). Outcome measures are, by contrast, seldom collected on a routine basis, with the exception of gross adverse outcome measures, for example still-birth rate and maternal mortality. With the widespread recognition that activity without good outcome is meaningless, increasing attention is now being paid to the methodological issues of measuring outcome. One problem is that any intervention may have a number of outcomes. Even for a procedure as simple as a herniorrhaphy, for example, one outcome could be an infected operative wound, another could be return to work within a defined period of time, another could be relief of the constant nagging aching pain, and another unexpected perioperative mortality. Sometimes the difference in perspective between physician and patient is so great that dissatisfaction is almost inevitable. For example, after a minor stroke the patient's hand often remains clumsy—a poor outcome for the patient, who will be dissatisfied. However, the patient's neurologist may know that there is no intervention that is going to alter that particular outcome, and his perspective is, perhaps, to succeed in helping the patient to stop smoking and to reduce his blood pressure. These are the best outcomes that the neurologist knows he can realistically achieve, even though they are not on the patient's agenda to any great extent.

One advance, which is only applicable to certain interventions, is to ask the patient what is most troubling him or her, and to relate the outcome to the most prominent symptom rather than to the disease process underlying that symptom. For example, a patient with varicose veins may complain either of the cosmetic disadvantage, or of aching pain in the legs, or of some other related symptom. If she rates the cosmetic impairment highly, then the outcome should be related to that rather than to other symptoms the relief of which is perhaps more easily measured. This innovative work from the University of Aberdeen is taking physicians back to their starting point—the relief of symptoms.[18] However, there are substantial methodological difficulties in measuring outcomes of interventions when there is a latency between the intervention and the outcome. For example, a patient who has a hip replacement may not gain the full benefit of that replacement until several months have passed. There are at present no regular systems for getting outcome measures in primary care practice linked back to the hospital record.

**Patient variables relating to satisfaction with care**

Patients vary in their propensity to be satisfied. Doctors and nurses know and recognise this, and speak in terms of 'good' (meaning compliant) patients and 'difficult' patients. Although undoubtedly there are individual variations in personality relating to patient satisfaction, some themes do emerge from the literature, so doctors know that extra efforts must be made to satisfy certain users. A meta-analysis of socio-demographic characteristics of patients as predictors of satisfaction has been performed by Hall and Dornan.[19] No overall relationship was found for sex, ethnicity, income or family size, but older people and less well educated people are significantly likely to be more satisfied. A patient

satisfaction scale specifically for older people had been construct-
ed by Cryns and colleagues.[20]

Some research suggests that patients who are dissatisfied with a
number of aspects of their life are also dissatisfied with their medical care;[21] in this perspective, dissatisfied patients are simply dissatisfied people. Of more immediate relevance to a physician's perspective is the strong research evidence that health status in itself is
related to satisfaction with care.[22,23] Hall, Feldstein and colleagues
found among older patients in a Health Maintenance Organisation that the more satisfied had better psychosocial health status.
Satisfaction was less strongly related to physical function and it was
not related to cognitive status. Although it is true that dissatisfaction in itself could cause a decline in health status (through a failure to comply with care or to return to care), it seems more prob-
able that, in the words of Hall and colleagues, sicker people are
unsatisfied people—a patient's overall outlook is coloured by ill
health. *A priori* this seems entirely reasonable: if the doctor cannot
get you better, then you may not be very satisfied. However, an
alternative hypothesis, proposed by Greenley and colleagues, is
that doctors react to sicker patients in ways that produce lower levels of satisfaction.[24] Hall has suggested that a physician, although
intrigued and stimulated by a difficult case, may often also find
such cases to be upsetting and frustrating, especially if no diagnosis can be made or if effective treatment is not available. Such
physician dissatisfaction is perceived by the patient who in turn is
also dissatisfied.

Physicians may make negative judgements about certain types of
patient, for example those who abuse alcohol. One study has asked
physicians directly how much they 'like' individual patients, and
related these ratings to the patient's health status.[25] As hypoth-
esised, physicians did like their healthier patients more, these
results being significant whether the measure of health status related to functional, social or emotional domains.

Anecdotal reports by patients with serious and progressive ill-
nesses towards death have described distress at how they have been
ignored by some doctors when 'nothing more can be done for
them'. A doctor who is less than competent at communicating support to a terminally ill patient may cause distress and dissatisfaction
by avoiding visits to the patient.

On a lighter note, there is no evidence to support the myth,
recounted to generations of medical students, that patients who
write down their symptoms on a piece of paper, or those who wear
tinted spectacles, are especially difficult to satisfy. There is, how-

ever, evidence that some systems of care will attract patients who are likely to be dissatisfied. Henryk-Gutt and Rees found that patients attending special migraine clinics showed high levels of hostility on the Minnesota Multiple Personality Inventory compared with a sample of other people with headaches.[26] Subsequent work by Fitzpatrick and myself showed that women who had themselves labelled their headaches as migraine (as opposed to tension headaches), who had initiated the referral to the migraine clinic themselves, who were rated anxious or depressed and who had had their symptoms for more than a year were particularly difficult to satisfy.[6,7]

It is important that such observations should not be taken as indicating that this cluster of patient characteristics is the patient's 'fault'. It rather means that physicians, forewarned by such knowledge, must take extra care in their attempts to impart information and express their care in a humane and empathic way.

### Physician variables relating to satisfaction with care

Doctors are just as various as patients. Some kind of 'specialty sorting' takes place during undergraduate education and postgraduate training, so that it may be hoped that doctors find themselves doing the kind of work for which they feel emotionally, psychologically and technically most suited. This is by no means always the case, and difficulties in finding a post in a preferred sub-specialty may lead a doctor to move to another less suited to his or her gifts. Chronically dissatisfied doctors are likely to have dissatisfied patients. Other doctors become 'burnt out' or clinically depressed, and patients readily perceive the diminution in effect referred to above. All this is experiential evidence. The more formal studies cited by Hall and Dornan indicate that patients are more satisfied with physicians in training than staff (consultant) physicians.[10] The authors cite studies indicating that younger physicians show more interpersonal and technical competence, and spend more time with their patients.

### Conclusions

In order to improve satisfaction with care, patients could change or doctors could change. Doctors must be responsive to the expectations of the community they serve, but patient satisfaction may be improved by the education of the community in relation to what it is reasonable to expect in terms of provision and accessibility of resources, and of what outcome it is technically possible to achieve. For many chronic disorders it is not possible to change significantly the biological impact of the disease, and it is unrealistic for a doctor to expect patients with these disorders to be satisfied with their lot, but they should be satisfied with their care, and it is here that doctors must do better. How can medical students and young doctors be educated and trained to preserve the enthusiasm and empathy with which they start? What psychological and other strategies can they adopt to avoid the routinisation of the consultation—something that is instantly perceived and resented by the patient?[27] What techniques can they adopt to impart information in an understandable form? How should they present choices to the patient? These are some of the challenges for those of us who educate the young people who will follow us.

## References

1. Richardson A, Charny M, Hanmer-Lloyd S. Public opinion and purchasing. *British Medical Journal* 1992; **304**: 680–2.
2. Klein R. On the Oregon trail: rationing health care. *British Medical Journal* 1991; **302**: 1–2.
3. Department of Health. *The patient's charter*. London: HMSO, 1991.
4. Hall JA, Roter DB, Katz NR. Meta-analysis of correlates of provider behaviour in medical encounters. *Medical Care* 1988; **26:** 657–75.
5. Davies AR, Ware JE. Involving consumers in quality of care assessment. *Health Affairs* 1988; **8**: 33–48.
6. Fitzpatrick R, Hopkins A. Patients' satisfaction with communication in neurological outpatient clinics. *Journal of Psychosomatic Research* 1981; **25**: 329–34.
7. Fitzpatrick R, Hopkins A. Referrals to neurologists for headaches not due to structural disease. *Journal of Neurology, Neurosurgery and Psychiatry* 1981; **44**: 1061–7.
8. Sox HC, Margulies I, Sox CM. Psychologically mediated effects of diagnostic tests. *Annals of Internal Medicine* 1981; **95**: 680–5.
9. Hartz AJ, Krakauer H, Young M, *et al.* Hospital characteristics and mortality rates. *New England Journal of Medicine* 1989; **321**: 1720–5.
10. Hall JA, Dornan MC. What patients think about their medical care, and how often they are asked: a meta-analysis of the satisfaction literature. *Social Science and Medicine* 1988, **27**: 935–9.
11. Roter DL, Hall JA. Studies of doctor-patient interaction. *Annual Review of Public Health* 1989; **10:** 163–80.
12. Fitzpatrick R, Hopkins A. Illness behaviour and headache, and the sociology of consultations for headache. In: Hopkins A, ed. *Headache: problems in diagnosis and management*. London: W. B. Saunders, 1988.
13. Raban J. *Hunting Mr Heartbreak*. London: Picador Press, 1992.
14. Hjortdahl P, Laerum E. Continuing of care in general practice: effect on patient satisfaction. *British Medical Journal* 1992; **304**: 1287–90.
15. Marquise MS, Davies AR, Ware JE. Patient satisfaction and change in

medical care provider: a longitudinal study. *Medical Care* 1983; **21**: 821–9.

16. Rossiter LF, Langwell K, Wan TTH, Rivnyak MS. Patient satisfaction among elderly enrollees and disenrollees in Medicare health maintenance organizations: results from the Medicare competition evaluation. *Journal of the American Medical Association* 1989; **262**: 57–63.

17. Hopkins A, ed. *Measures of the quality of life, and the uses to which such measures may be put.* London: RCP Publications, 1992.

18. Ruta D. University of Aberdeen, personal communication, 1992.

19. Hall JA, Dornan MC. Patient sociodemographic characteristics as predictors of satisfaction with medical care: a meta-analysis. *Social Science and Medicine* 1990; **30**: 811–8.

20. Cryns AG, Nichols RC, Katz LA, Calkins E. The hierarchical structure of geriatric patient satisfaction: an older patient satisfaction scale designed for HMOs. *Medical Care* 1989; **27**: 802–16.

21. Roberts RE, Pascoe GC, Attkisson CC. Relationship of service satisfaction to life satisfaction and perceived well-being. *Evaluation and Program Planning* 1983; **6**: 373–83.

22. Pascoe GC. Patient satisfaction in primary health care: a literature review and analysis. *Evaluation and Program Planning* 1983; **6**: 185.

23. Hall JA, Feldstein M, Fretwell MD, Rowe JW, Epstein AM. Older patients' health status and satisfaction with care in an HMO population. *Medical Care* 1990; **28**: 261–70.

24. Greenley JR, Young TB, Schoenherr RA. Psychological distress and patient satisfaction. *Medical Care* 1982; **20**: 373–85.

25. Hall J, Epstein AM, De Ciantis ML, McNeil BJ. Physicians' liking for their patients: more evidence for the role of affect in medical care. *Health Psychology* 1993; **12**: 141–7.

26. Henryk-Gutt R, Rees WL. Psychological aspects of migraine. *Journal of Psychosomatic Research* 1973; **17**: 141–53.

27. Bloor M. Professional autonomy and client exclusion: a case study in ENT clinics. In: Wadsworth M, Robinson D, eds. *Studies in everyday medical life.* London: Martin Robertson, 1976.

*Note added in proof*

The Royal College of Physicians will in 1993 be publishing a report *Communication in medicine.*

A further useful reference is: Roter DL, Hall JA. *Doctors talking with patients/Patients talking with doctors.* Westport CT: Auburn House, 1992.

# 9 | The consumer's preference

**Linda Lamont**
*The Patients Association, London*

### The missing link

One of my favourite American cartoons shows a heavily bandaged man in a hospital bed. His anxious looking wife is saying: 'Dear, I've looked up your insurance and you are covered for falling off the garage roof but not for hitting the ground'.

The average American consumer has become expert at spotting the gaps in health cover in a system where a major consideration in changing jobs is the level of health insurance that the new employer offers. Will our own internal market mean that people need to know the length of the local health district's waiting lists for operations and whether the local fundholding general practice will accept them, before they decide to move?

League tables for various aspects of cost, quality and performance are already used by managers and health professionals for their own purposes, but consumer satisfaction is not yet regarded as a key outcome measure. Nor could it be, without national standards and accepted methods of measurement to set against them. Perhaps in future we will be able to refer to a consumer rating chart to see how one's local health services compare with others.

Patients cannot say how satisfied they are with the health services they receive unless they know the standards that they have a reasonable right to expect, the choices that are available, and how these compare with what is on offer elsewhere.* Access to such a range of information would not sound an impossible request in the context of other types of service such as travel or even education, yet it is apparently for consumers of health services.

Health providers are making assorted attempts at measuring patient satisfaction, as they are required to do, but there is as yet

---

*'What do patients have a right to expect?' was the subject of the first Dame Elizabeth Ackroyd Symposium, held in honour of the Patients Association's late chairperson in May 1991.

no central consumer agency that seeks to measure standards uniquely from the patient's point of view. Individual patients seek help and advice from a number of organisations such as Community Health Councils, self-help groups and national charities like the Patients Association.

## Why people are dissatisfied: the communication gap

One way of understanding current dissatisfaction with health services is to look at the sort of complaints that people bring to an organisation like the Patients Association, and through them to identify some gaps and problems in the system. For example, a consistent element in most of the complaints we receive is about communication, or the lack of it.

Poor communication was an important theme in the complaints picked out by the Health Service Commissioner in 1991: 'I wonder how those complained about would feel if they received such inadequate services themselves. A better understanding of patients' worries must be learned by National Health Service staff'.[1]

Meredith, in an impressive survey, rates communication as '. . . the most significant issue of dissatisfaction . . . confirmed by successive studies of patients' experiences of hospital care, utilising a range of methods'.[2] Difficulties in communication are also a consistent, if often underlying, theme of patients' complaints about general practice. The availability of suitable information, and when or how it is presented to them, affects patients' perception of the quality of health care they receive. But it is difficult to isolate communication from other aspects of poor performance, as demonstrated by the General Medical Council's proposals for the review of professional performance.[3]

## Policy and performance: the information gap

'Buzz words for one audience can be gobbledegook for another' said Sir Roy Griffiths at his Audit Commission Management Lecture in 1991. He illustrated this by remarking that the division between purchasing and the provision of health care was not understood by, or indeed interesting to, the man in the street. It may be true that patients' interests tend to be centred on the services they actually receive rather than the policy decisions involved, but they need to understand in outline major changes in organisation such as the purchaser/provider split and contracting, if they are to comment productively on their satisfaction with the services they receive.

The proposed plan to set up regional National Health Service (NHS) information centres is to be welcomed. It is in the interests of policy makers to share with the public in clear terms how they plan to provide health services, including hard choices that have to be made about priorities. They should not assume that people are incapable of rational thought. Millions of pounds were spent by the Department of Health on a leaflet for every household, explaining the reorganisation of the NHS. The content was patronising in tone and illustration, contained little hard information, and said practically nothing about consumer involvement in the process. There had obviously not been any consultation with those who actually work with patients, or with patients themselves.

However, some regions are making a serious effort to find out what consumers think. South West Thames Regional Health Authority (RHA) used information from clients, carers and voluntary bodies to inform the players in a three-day simulation exercise (Kaleidoscope) in May 1991 to act out how community care plans might work in practice. Although it seems that consumers were not directly involved, this is an improvement on East Anglia RHA's similar simulation exercise, 'Rubber Windmill', where they were not involved at all.[4]

North West Thames RHA has commissioned a mammoth survey of 10,000 adults by comprehensive personal interviews ranging over eight key variables, including consumer satisfaction with local health services. Such a survey could be of tremendous value to the region in deciding future policy. Personal interviews of this kind, however non-directive, will also have positive results for at least some of those interviewed, in terms of increased awareness of the availability of local health services and of health promotion issues like diet, exercise, smoking and drinking.

An initial survey of the National Association of Health Authorities and Trusts database of contracts shows an interesting variety of interpretations by Health Authorities of their brief to include patient satisfaction surveys as a way of monitoring their services. Examples range from a token clause to a detailed set of specifications for survey and complaints procedures.

Taylor, in his report for the King's Fund on research in primary care, hopes that '. . . any future work of the Primary Care Development Fund might most desirably focus more directly on consumers' expectations and the end-point outcomes of the care they receive, rather than analysing mainly the activities of its providers'.[5]

The need for consumer audit emerges also as a major quality issue in the report commissioned by the Management Executive on the future role of the Family Health Service Authority (FHSA) in the new NHS structure.[6] In an appendix to the report, FHSAs are urged to support targeted and in-depth studies of patients' views rather than quick questionnaire surveys, since quality improvement in general practitioners' performance is more likely to be achieved through constructively critical feedback.

Discussion of the role of consumer audit is remarkable for its absence from the paper issued at the same time by the Management Executive on 'Integrating primary and secondary health care'. Apart from a fleeting reference to 'patient-responsive services' on the first page, there is no discussion as to how patients' satisfaction with services is to be monitored. Is this an example of a buzz word being used as a substitute for serious planning?

In recent years, the Department of Health has added the Patients Association to its list of those to be consulted when issuing new circulars. This was originally, I believe, an exercise in tokenism, but I like to think that the exercise is beginning to be taken more seriously. For example, when we were consulted about draft circulars on procedures for hospital discharge and consent to treatment, we were able to use our knowledge of patients' concerns about these subjects to make practical suggestions for the implementation of policy. As a result of this process we are also in a better position to advise patients about correct procedures. In the same way, guidance about the Access to Medical Records Act (1991) included for the first time a model information leaflet for patients as concrete evidence of similar consultation with consumers at the draft stage. The Association's position as a reference point between the Department and individual patients who come to us with complaints or problems means that we can provide information to both. There are of course many other health consumer organisations that could do the same.

### Expectations of patients and doctor: the reality gap

'Promises, promises': that is likely to be the wry reaction of patients who are on long waiting lists or sitting for hours in an outpatient clinic, should they happen to read one of the optimistic mission statements being dispensed by their health region or hospital. It is more likely that most patients will never read such a document.

The new chairman of South Western RHA rushed out a health charter (1990) which was said to have caused mild apoplexy among his staff and Community Health Councils when they read it. The staff wondered how they could deliver such promises; the Community Health Councils complained that they had not been consulted. On the other hand, South West Thames RHA, in designing their 'Ten golden rules' wall-chart, wisely expressed their mission in terms of 'should' rather than 'will', thus making it a question of intentions and not promises. Always lingering in the wings is the major caveat '. . . as the budget allows'.

Warrington Health Authority have produced a more practical document in their patient/staff charter, which recognises that the information requirements of patients and staff are not necessarily the same, even though the end result desired by both is a good service. They try to tackle a broad range of services, including the care of terminally ill patients and those suffering from AIDS, but they have still to work out how they will incorporate any information about patient satisfaction into staff training.

The Charter for Children in Hospital designed by the National Association for Children in Hospital (NAWCH) is used by Warrington Health Authority as a standard for their children's services. The NAWCH (now Action for Sick Children) charter is widely admired in Britain and abroad as setting a reasonable standard backed by detailed research and consultation with both clinicians and managers as well as patients or their parents. It is a model for other work by patients' and users' organisations in trying to establish realistic standards of care in specific areas.

Some of the broader-based statements of patients' rights run the double risk of raising expectations unrealistically for the patient and of being ignored by health professionals as unworkable. A delicate balance is required between statements of principle and practical methods by which good service can be achieved. Cancerlink produced in 1990 a Declaration of Rights for people with cancer which we often send to patients. This is a statement of broad principle which it is hoped will provoke enough patient and professional feedback to go to the next stage of providing more detailed specifications of what patients need.

Patients need to know what they have a right to expect before they can comment on the quality of the services they actually receive. The much heralded Patient's Charter lists the remarkably few rights that patients have, including some with significant qualification.[7] For example, the right to a second opinion was described as subject to the agreement of the general practitioner, but it is the difficulty in obtaining this agreement that is often the subject of complaint.

Much of what is contained in the charter is a summary of

existing good practice, including three 'new' rights. One of these, the right to a prompt reply from the Chief Executive or General Manager of a provider unit, does not necessarily ensure any specific action in response to a complaint. The major emphasis in the Patient's Charter is on acute services and on waiting times for elective surgery. The rights of people who need long-term care and services in the community are hardly addressed. It is in primary and community care services that more work needs to be done on patient satisfaction. How the local patients' charters to be produced by individual health authorities will tackle these areas remains to be seen.

Meanwhile the doctors who treat us continue to work within what some of their own profession describe as a feudal system. Anyone who has received hospital treatment will have observed the cohort of staff surrounding the consultant in a pyramidal and defensive structure. A kind of Stonehenge of organisational monoliths protects the consultant from too much direct personal contact with the patient, who should only speak when spoken to and then to say what the consultant wants to hear. Of course this is not true of everyone, but we are told about this attitude too often by patients to believe that such behaviour is exceptional. Yet how much of this frustration felt by patients comes through in surveys of satisfaction?

When patients do express dissatisfaction with the outcome of their treatment, doctors will often complain that patients' expectations of what can be done to alleviate their condition are unrealistic. In this case, the doctor has obviously not explained carefully enough what he can and cannot do. It is in the doctor's own interests to dispel the image of a magician.

'The medical profession inhabits a secret garden', said Lord Dainton, introducing the Chapel Hill conference of British and American medical experts in May 1990.[8] As the sole speaker representing patients' interests, I felt privileged to be allowed inside. Lord Dainton was right in describing the public's perception of doctors as being of an inward looking group who often do not seem to understand that their patients' health is interrelated with many other factors. People do not live in a compartmentalised way, any more than a diseased organ or a broken limb can be treated in isolation from the rest of the body.

One of the most important long-term remedies for patient dissatisfaction with the general attitudes of doctors is to improve medical training. The General Medical Council in its annual report for 1990 rightly identifies two essential aims in improving basic medical education as: 'to reduce the awesome factual overload that still characterises most curricula, and to promote a much greater degree of self-motivated learning than they currently feature'. It is a pity that increased attention to communication skills was not listed as at least the third essential arm, though it does appear elsewhere in the report.

Happily some medical schools are aware of the problem. Several now emphasise the need for evidence of communication skills, voluntary work experience and a mature personality in the candidates they choose. Leicester runs a Man (*sic*) and Society programme which examines how social institutions like family and work can affect health. St Bartholomew's and Birmingham Medical Schools are both investing real money in improving the communication skills of doctors and nurses. Communication aspects of general practice training are a major component of the Oxford Practice Skills Project.

## What is needed to bridge the gaps?

Accurate consumer feedback must be based on better information for the general public and training for those who represent their interests. If consumer auditors are to be accepted as valid partners by health professionals and managers, they have to be seen to be knowledgeable about the basic processes of the health system. A core qualification, possibly in information about health services obtained through the open learning process, would help to give them credibility.

There are several communication channels already in existence which can be developed further to improve the productive exchange of information and ideas between health professionals, managers and patients. A number of the Royal Colleges now have patient liaison groups. The United Kingdom Central Council for Nursing, Midwifery and Health Visiting has set up formal links with consumer organisations.

From the consumer side, the Patients Association has organised a Quality Assurance for Patients group to which doctors and managers have been invited. Our Patients Forum has now been running for more than two years and has regular meetings at which national organisations representing a wide spectrum of patients' interests share current concerns with each other and with experts in the field such as the Health Ombudsman and the Audit Commission.

The methods used for making surveys of patient satisfaction

must obviously be flexible enough to be relevant in different situations. Fitzpatrick suggests that patient participation groups or tape
recordings of patients' descriptions of their experience may be
valuable for staff.[9] Newcastle Health Authority has found such
groups useful for getting patients in hospital to express their views
more freely. Other chapters in this book describe other methods.

When surveys are being planned, crucial questions have to be
asked about the reasons for doing the survey in the first place, its
reliability and validity, and whether those who commissioned it are
prepared to act on the results. Selected respondents could be
asked to join a small hospital or practice management group to
discuss complaints and comments in more depth over a modest
meal. American hospitals find this attracts patients to respond; it
also produces welcome feedback material. Response rates to surveys might also be increased by the introduction of a 'lucky number' scheme, the respondent whose survey form was drawn being
eligible for a prize.

Complaints are a rich source of material for identifying areas of
concern which do not necessarily surface as a result of a standard
questionnaire. This seems more obvious to those of us who work in
the health consumer field than to managers or health professionals. Yet a close examination of the wound will produce a better
result than sticking a plaster over it.

Better information for patients is a major factor in improving
satisfaction. The explosion in self-help groups at local and national
level demonstrates people's need for more support and their will-
ingness to help each other. The information materials that such
groups produce could be much better used, were they of a sufficient standard. If a fraction of the money being spent on information technology for doctors and managers were to be offered to
patients' organisations, spectacular improvements could be seen in
terms of well informed customers.

Those who give out information could provide a parallel function of analysing the problems and queries that are brought to
them. The Patients Association has devised a database which can
do just this and which could in principle be used by other organisations. On a large scale it could help to provide useful information
about outcomes. As health management and accountability
processes become more complex, the consumer/patient needs
proper representation more than ever before. If providers of
health services, whether doctors or managers, really want to
improve outcomes in terms of patients' satisfaction, they will welcome better organised consumer representation. This will mean

involving consumers in the setting of standards, monitoring the delivery of services, and measuring outcomes, including quality of life issues, as well as agreeing priorities when budgets are limited. The NHS Management Executive has recently published a paper on consultation with consumers ('Local voices') which makes an effort to address the problem. Consumer organisations have also been thinking through the most practical ways in which their voices can be taken into account by managers (Involving the Community, NCC).

Meanwhile the Clinical Standards Advisory Group has no consumer representatives as members or observers, even though it is generally agreed that an element of consumer feedback has a place in the medical audit process.

One way forward would be the formation of a Health Consumer Standards Board which would provide an accredited channel for considering consumers' satisfaction or dissatisfaction with the standard of services they received. Such a body would work in conjunction with the professional organisations, together with an independent inspectorate and existing bodies like the Audit Commission and the Health Commissioner.

## References

1. Health Service Commissioner. *Report (October 1990 to March 1991)*. London: HMSO, 1991.
2. Meredith P. Audit and the quality of clinical care: patient satisfaction. *Annals of the Royal College of Surgeons of England* (College and Faculty Bulletin) 1992; **73**: 51–4.
3. General Medical Council. *Performance review procedures* (Draft). London: GMC, 1992.
4. East Anglia Regional Health Authority. *Contracting for health outcomes*. Report of the 'Rubber Windmill' exercise, 1990.
5. Taylor D. *Developing primary care: opportunities for the 1990s*. Research report 10. London: King's Fund Institute, 1991.
6. Foster A. *FHSAs: today's and tomorrow's priorities*. York Regional Health Authority, 1991.
7. Department of Health. *The patient's charter*. London: HMSO, 1991.
8. Lord Dainton. Opening the secret garden. In: *Health care provision under financial constraint: a decade of change*. L'Etang H, ed. London: Royal Society of Medicine Services, 1990.
9. Fitzpatrick R. Surveys of patient satisfaction. 1. Important general considerations. *British Medical Journal* 1991; **302**: 887–9.

## RCP paperbacks

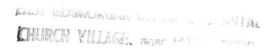